ADVANCE PRAISE FOR *NOTES LEFT BEHIND*

"Elena has left behind a story of resilience, hope and most of all, love. We can't help but take her into our hearts, and carry the best of her into our lives."

—Jeffrey Zaslow, coauthor of *The Last Lecture*

"This is a stunning story that teaches us how precious children, family and life are, and that the sacrifices we make are worth it. I won't forget the Desserich family, and neither will you."

—James Patterson, bestselling author

"My heart goes out to them . . . but I have to admire the way they were able to teach Elena to see her life as joyful, and not as a tragedy. They really are inspiring parents."

—Susan Wagner, AOL's ParentDish.com

notes left behind

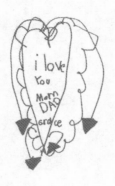

notes left behind

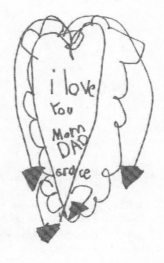

Brooke and Keith Desserich

WILLIAM MORROW
An Imprint of HarperCollins*Publishers*

HarperCollins books may be purchased for educational, business, or sales promotional
use. For information please write: Special Markets Department, HarperCollins Publishers, 10 East 53rd Street, New York, NY 10022.

Designed by Lisa Stokes

Library of Congress Cataloging-in-Publication Data has been applied for.

ISBN 978-0-06-188639-3

09   10   11   12   13   OV/RRD   10   9   8   7   6   5   4   3

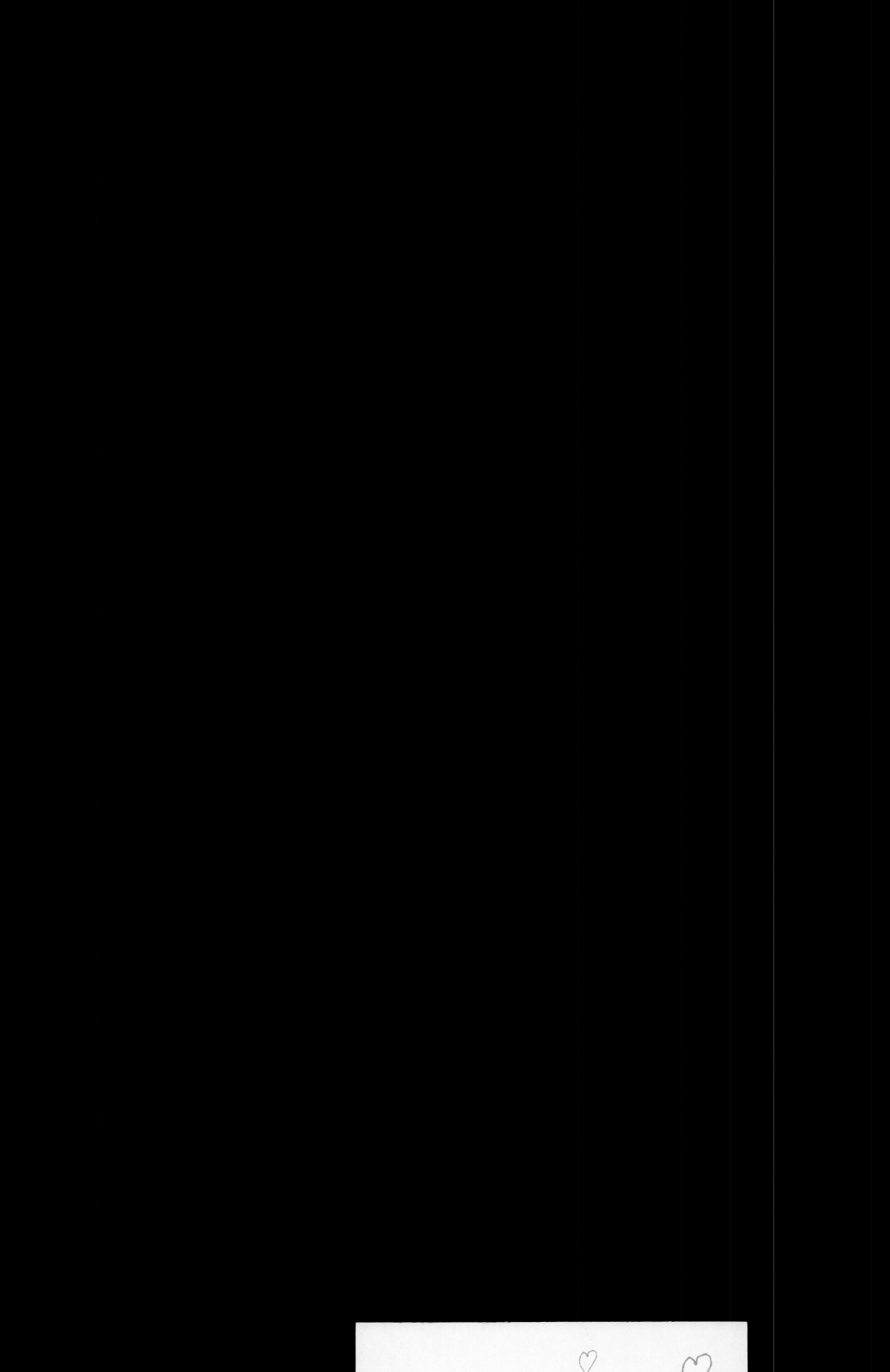

THIS IS OUR ELENA

She always eats her vegetables first.

She can never wear enough pink.

She always writes her name backward—not because she doesn't know how to write it, but because she "just likes the way it looks."

She crosses her legs when she sits.

There is nothing better than art class, except, of course, a trip to the library.

Fiction is better than nonfiction.

Skip the pop, give her milk. And pour it in a wineglass and say "cheers."

She loves "squibble-squabbles" (lace and ruffles).

Tights are best when in jungle patterns or polka dots.

No pants, only dresses.

She loves babies.

When you play school, she is always the teacher.

Mom is best for cuddling.

Sally (a grumpy old Chihuahua) is the best pet she never had.

You can never have enough headbands.

All she ever wants in life is to be a mom.

She is simple. She is our Elena.

To learn more about Elena's story,
visit www.notesleftbehind.com.

contents

from the authors

B ROOKE HAS HER NOTE. I have mine. They are tucked
away in our briefcases, always with us, never out of reach. I
found mine in the black backpack that we took to Elena's wish
trip. On the cover of the envelope is a lopsided purple heart, just
the way Elena drew them best. On the side she wrote "DAD" in
clear pink letters before sealing the envelope and hiding it in the
hidden pouch of the backpack. Brooke found her letter in the
side pocket of her briefcase, where Elena had put it many months
before. Hers too is in an envelope, with "MOM" carefully spelled
out in the unsteady handwriting Elena had as the paralysis slowly
set in. These are two of many letters that Elena hid for us in the
last nine months of her life, some hidden between books on the
bookshelf, in the corners of our dresser drawers, between dishes
in the china cabinet or between photos stacked away in boxes
during the construction, each note deliberately left professing her
love for her family. They are constant reminders of her determi-

nation and her inspiration. She knew somehow that one day we would need them to continue.

I love the heart on my letter. I yearn for her handwritten "DAD" that is written not only on my envelope but on everything from printer paper to scraps of paper around the house. Still, I can't get beyond the envelope. The last of Elena's letters that I read told me she was sorry she was sick. I found this letter in the drawer by my bedside two weeks after her death. I cried for the week following. I can only imagine what this letter says. Maybe it tells me she knew more than we could ever imagine, that from her original diagnosis with brain cancer to the end she understood. She understood the concealed conversations with the doctors, she understood that she would never regain what she lost and she understood that it would ultimately take her life. But most of all, I hope that she understood that we loved her too. I only wish I had left her notes in return.

This book too is a note from Elena, messages from a little girl who taught our family so much about life. And although written in our hand, it represents the lessons of a six-year-old girl in the only way she knew to tell them to us: through her heart. In truth, these lessons were always intended for her sister, Gracie. They will always continue to be for Gracie. Sitting with Elena that fateful November night with the lights of the IV monitor illuminating her soft features and warm smile, I knew that our lives would be forever changed. It happened the moment they told us that she had 135 days to live. Thankfully we had more, and in the nine months that followed, Elena would grow wise and tired, we as parents would become fearless and Gracie would lose her best friend—her "Lena." Yet Gracie was still too young to understand and remember. The journal was my way of

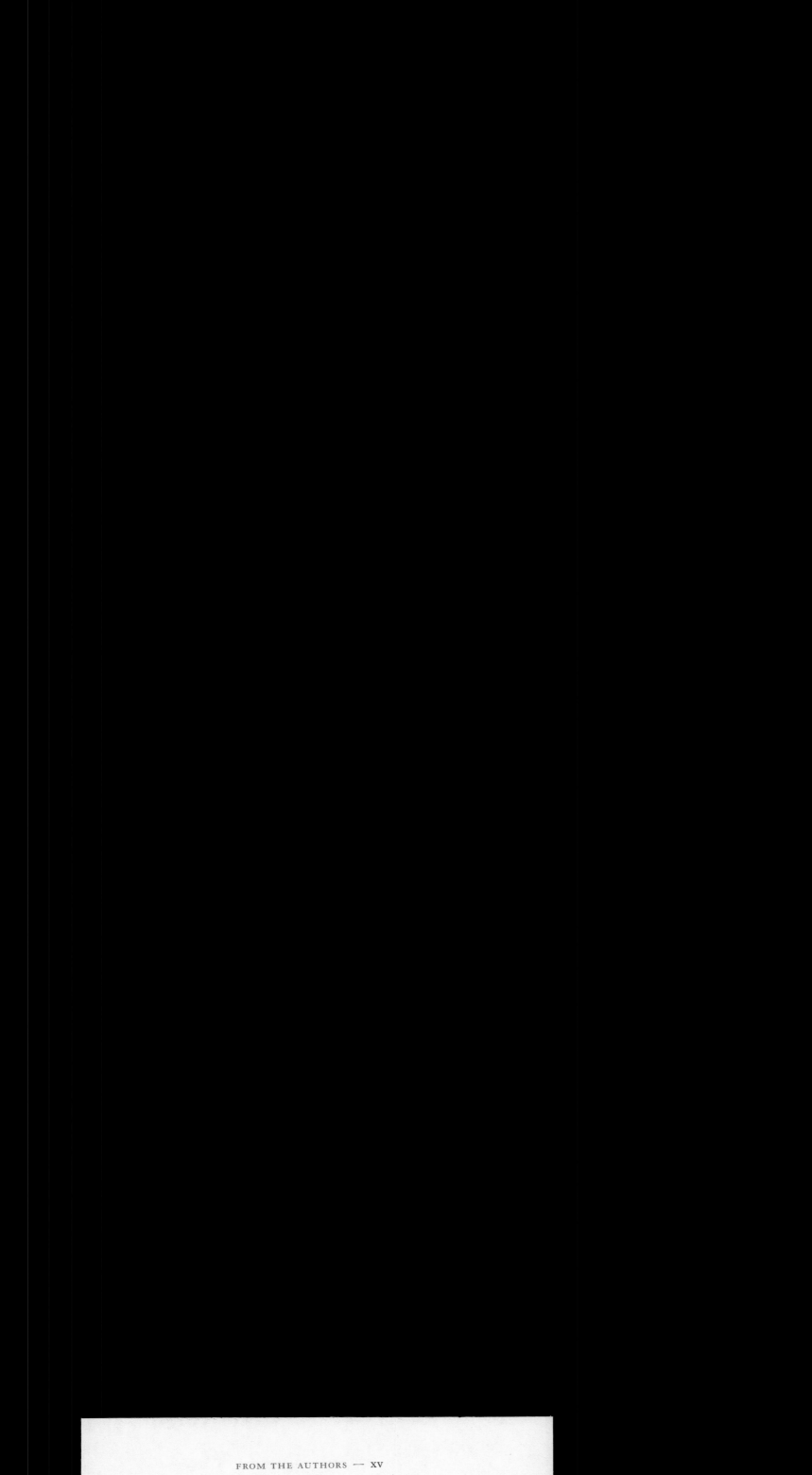

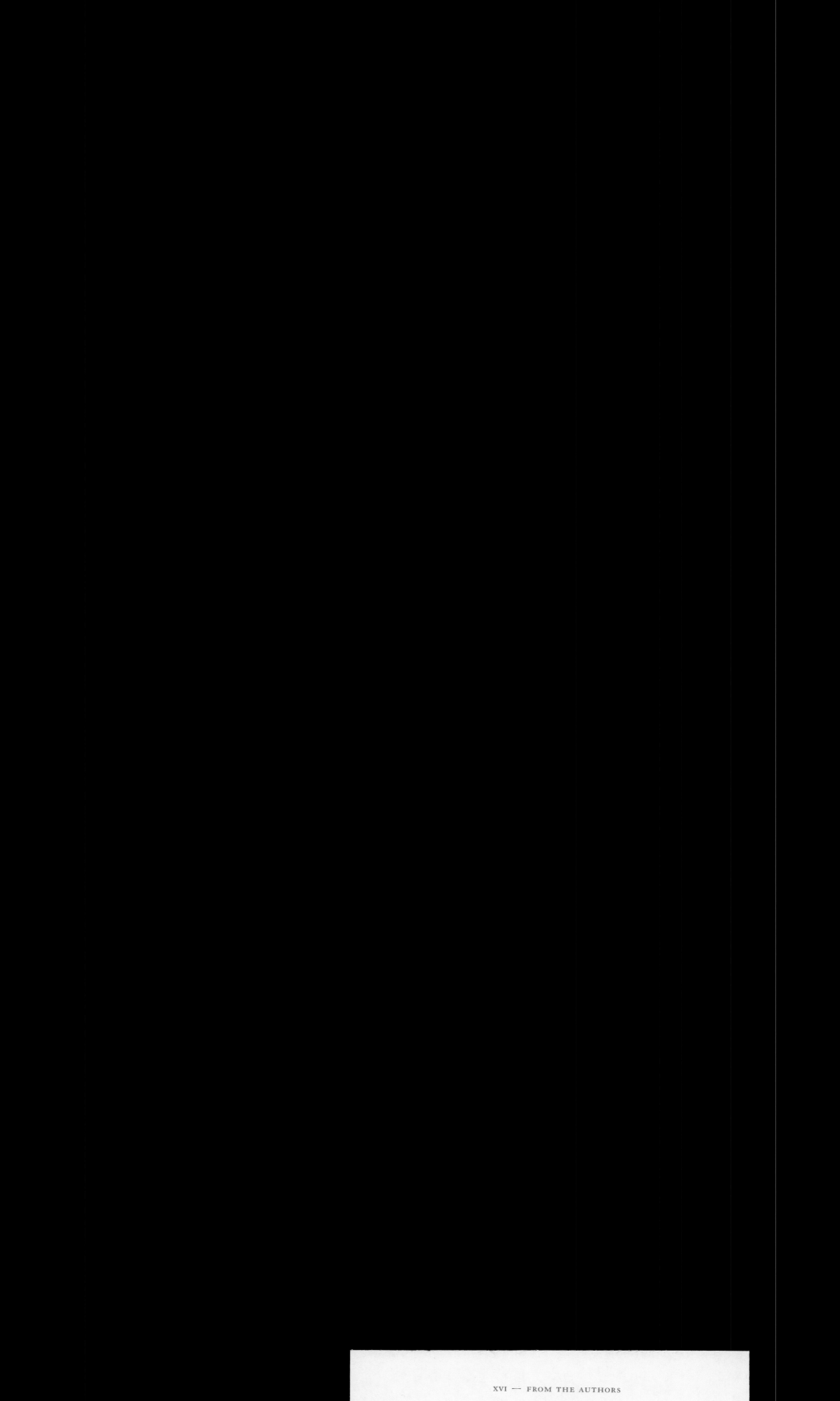

notes left behind

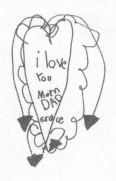

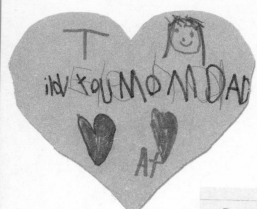

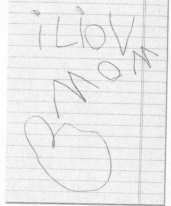

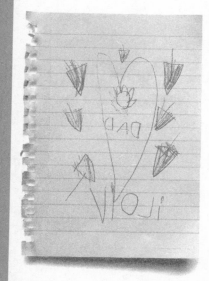

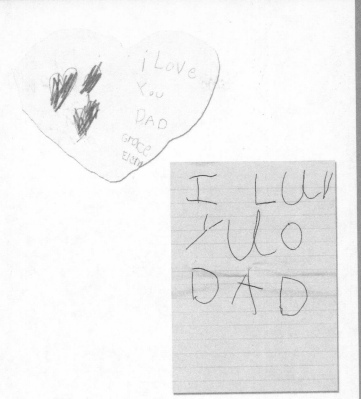

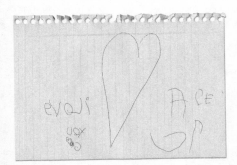

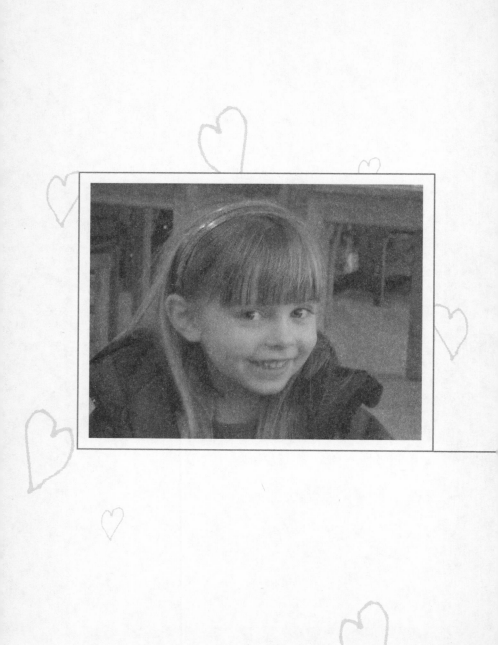

part 1: the beginning

I T BEGAN EARLY. We called it "binner." With her IV sur-gery scheduled for 7 A.M., the last time she could eat was 1 in the morning. So at midnight I woke her up to a breakfast/ dinner of yogurt—except the nurse forgot to order yogurt before the kitchen closed and we ended up with a meal of pudding and applesauce instead. From 1 A.M. to dawn we talked about "Alice in Wonderland," her new discovery of the TV remote and what she always wanted to do. And although I couldn't always under-stand her words because of the tumor, I could usually under-stand her drawings.

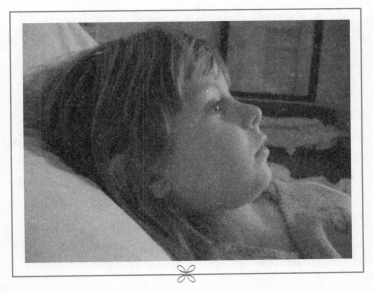

First came a circle with squiggly lines. This was where she wanted to go—the only problem was that I did not know what she was telling me. After several tries and more than enough frustration on her part, I figured out that she was talking about the "little restaurant"—the chili parlor a mile from our house. With this her face lit up as she told me she wanted spaghetti and cheese. This was a remarkably simple request and we added it to the list. The next one was a bit harder: the Eiffel Tower. To this day, I still don't know where she came up with this one. Regardless, this was the list and what we needed to accomplish. From there the list continued to the "street of dresses," which I immediately recognized as a wedding dress district in our town, but I feigned ignorance. It was the same street I had deliberately driven down on the way home with the girls for the past five years, while telling them to pick out their dresses. Now she was asking me to take her to the same shops that I had always envisioned taking her to when she was engaged. Now I questioned if she would ever make it that far. Still, it went on the list.

As the night went on, we continued to talk. She wanted to talk and I wanted to listen. Sleep was not as important as it was three days ago. I watched her face illuminated by the lights on the heart monitor wondering if I would remember every detail: the softness of her cheeks, the dancing glow of her eyes, the innocence of her thoughts. But was it all a nightmare? Would I awake tomorrow and the tumor would simply be gone? Maybe this was just a lesson from life and by tomorrow the tumor would miraculously disappear. I could only hope.

That night, the doctors sent us home for rest, but after they told us that our daughter had only 135 days to live, sleep wasn't in

our plans. Still we smiled, wiped the tears from our eyes and tried
to pretend that everything was all right. But it was Elena who
had the best suggestion. Before leaving, she wanted to celebrate
Christmas. So we took time to carefully find her precious Jesus
and angel ornaments and hang them on the tree that the grandparents had hastily put up only minutes before. Ironic, because in
previous years, I'd always insisted on not putting up the tree before
December 15. Still, this year it couldn't come soon enough.

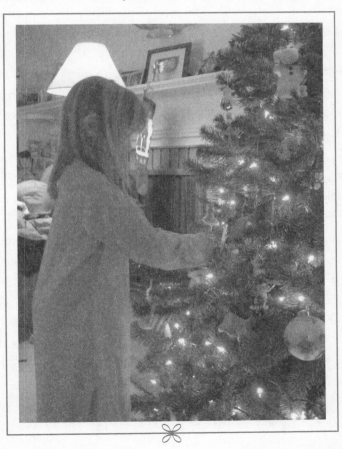

Brooke read the girls a book before bed. It was the longest book we could find.

Day 2—NOVEMBER 30

The trip to Memphis was a long one. Elena has been accepted into a program there, offering experimental brain stem treatments, so we booked the first flight out. God love Elena and her desire to be pretty. To protect her from sickness, we took all of the necessary precautions, from air scrubbing and cleaning the home to getting flu shots for the entire family. Lastly, we brought dust masks from the hospital to have Elena wear on the plane. She would have none of this. Of course, she did appreciate being wheeled around in a wheelchair like a queen on a throne, but to wear a dust mask was just too much. After all, how would her fellow passengers feel about her looks? After much prompting and prodding, we both ended up wearing masks. She said I looked silly.

Airline clearance was another issue. With Elena and her drugs, it took a good hour to get through security. It took another hour to get Mom past all the gift shops. Whatever Elena wanted, she got, as Mom caved and bought her a new Beanie Baby and ice cream. If we had passed any more gift shops through the terminal, I'm certain we would have gone broke.

Two hours later we were in Memphis. There we were introduced to the new hospital and our new regimen. Contrary to previous conversations, the pace was fast as Elena received the attention she needed to give us a fighting chance. Before the evening was out, we had had four consultations lasting over one hour each, two X-rays, an orientation and a new home. She was exhausted and so was I. We ended the evening in the hotel room reading the get-well cards written by her classmates from kindergarten. She crawled into bed clutching the cards beneath the covers. I'm still trying to figure out how to get them away from her before she falls asleep.

So far, so good. Two days into our time and we've met all the right people. We've even taken care of two of Elena's wishes—to put up the Christmas tree and go to the airport.

Day 3—DECEMBER 1

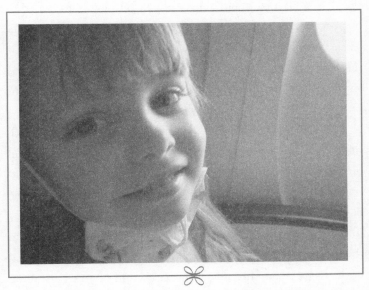

For the first time, we saw a picture of the tumor. It's not only large, but concealed within the walls of Elena's brain stem. The prognosis isn't good. Originally, we were told that we would have three to six months. It's little reassurance that now the doctors say possibly seven months to over a year. That's still not enough time to see my baby's driving lessons, first date, wedding or children. The milestones that we remember most in life have been ripped from her hands. No chance, no hope. But it's still months and right now anything is better than what we were originally told.

Elena's getting very tired now and has developed a fear of anyone with blue gloves. After all, these are the same hands that poked and prodded her for the past week. I think she fears the gloves over the shots at this point. I'm thinking of buying a pack of clear gloves for the doctors in her wing just to calm her anxiety. She's also started to listen and ask questions. I've always known that Elena listened to our conversations, but now she's added to her vocabulary words such as "IV flushing," "MRI" and "CT scan." Somehow I always knew she would learn about all of this if she ever decided to become a doctor, but I never imagined she would be getting this education as a patient. But now she listens intently while I try to conceal the truth of what we face.

Tonight we decided to treat her to a dinner of her choice with her cousins, who drove up from Alabama to visit. It was a good idea at the time, but by the time we ended her doctors' appointments at 7 P.M., it was a bit late. As a result, while she enjoyed the balloon art hat that we had made for her, Elena didn't make it far into the meal before she fell asleep on her aunt's shoulder. From there her fatigue only contributed to her condition and we ended up having to carry her out of the restaurant or risk her falling over her own feet. I know she needs the company, but right now I think she also needs the rest. She has had a rough week and it's just the beginning.

Day 4—DECEMBER 2

Today was a good day. It was Saturday and we didn't have to go to the hospital—all we had to do was make Elena smile. She was tired this morning, but also very hungry for waffles. After waking up at 6 A.M. from her open-eyed and teeth-gnawing sleep, all she wanted was waffles with butter. At first we couldn't understand her with her limited voice, but thank goodness she could at least spell "WFL" to communicate her wishes. She had to have waffles with whipped cream, chocolate chips and cherries for eyes. And except for the cherries, she ate the entire thing. Must be the steroids working.

For the first time, Elena has now lost sensation in her thighs. Now she has a limp in her right leg, no gag reflex, limited ability in her right arm, loss of left-eye peripheral vision and reduced sensation in her legs. I know this because in an attempt to raise a smile, I tried to tickle her most ticklish part: her knees. It used to be that all I needed to do was motion toward her knees and I would instantaneously get a wide-mouth smile. Now she simply looks at me with annoyance. I miss tickling my little girl. For a dad, it's always about more than horseplay—it's a way of expressing my love. I'll just have to find another way to make her smile.

Day 5—DECEMBER 3

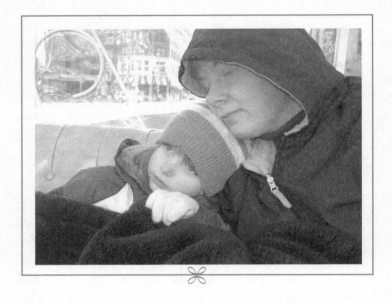

A horse-drawn carriage ride was her third choice after the "little restaurant" and the Eiffel Tower. (I think part of it was because when we read "Alice in Wonderland" that first night we skipped past "Cinderella" and an illustration of the pumpkin carriage.) Luckily, Memphis had plenty of them. So in the face of 20-degree wind chills, we made our way downtown to catch a horse-drawn carriage ride. Instantly, the smile came back through the strain of anxiety that had recently robbed my little girl's face. It was back and I felt like a father again as we roamed the streets. In the face of cancer I could make her smile and I could give her back the childhood that she was about to lose. And while it was bitterly cold, Elena's smile was enough to warm all of our hearts. I hope this will be a lasting memory.

From there, we went to the stuffed animal factory to create a bear of her choosing. Although one of her requests, this was far less satisfying for both of us in the Christmas rush. Packed into a store, we found nearly one hundred Christmas shoppers vying for first place in the commercialized race against time. And for the first time, I was jealous. I was jealous of their joy, jealous of their ignorance, jealous of their rushing. I wanted to be the one more concerned about getting to the next store rather than struggling to lock away every memory of a conceivably limited future.

But then, I realized that my family and I were the ones who truly appreciated the season and all that it meant. You see, Elena's illness has taught us to squeeze the very last sunlight out of every day and to see our children as more than just a Christmas list. And while I certainly still don't desire this lesson, I will never squander another day again. I think Elena also realized this and instead asked to leave the mall and get an ice cream cone. We proceeded to leave, of course, after having convinced Gracie, who already had her eyes on a ballerina outfit for her stuffed poodle.

What does all of this mean? I don't know and I don't think that every moment demands a lesson. All I know is that these memories need to last. Whether we go to the Eiffel Tower or to the grocery store, they both can be treasured moments if you make the most of them.

Day 6—DECEMBER 4

Today was Elena's birthday. Not really, but close enough. With the radiation treatments and biopsy happening this Wednesday, today was close enough for her grandparents and us. So after her morning appointments, we all headed off to lunch and then back to the room for presents. There she opened a guitar from her aunt and a digital camera from Grandma and Grandpa. Now we have pictures from her point of view. Too bad that every picture she takes is from the waist down.

Day 8—DECEMBER 6

Last night we faced one big heart-wrenching decision. In the end, we decided that the two-week delay in treating Elena's tumor was more than we were willing to risk. With her mouth now paralyzed and her inability to swallow, we feared that waiting another two weeks for a biopsy would just be too much. Our hopes are that in treating this now with radiation, we will be able to recover many of her normal functions for the recovery period.

About midway through the day today, I noticed Elena was getting very quiet. I asked her what was wrong and she told me she was getting mad that everyone was talking about her and around her and no one was talking *to* her. This is the new challenge. So I asked the doctors and nurses to talk directly to her, all while not going too far. We explained what will happen with radiation and how everything we are doing now will help her to get home and back to normal. We have a long six weeks ahead of us, but I think as the radiation begins, we will settle into our routine and she will start feeling better.

The prognosis has not changed, and we are still looking for a miracle, but we have found tentative comfort in making a decision and moving forward to make Elena better. Though we still feel the anger and sadness, we force ourselves to stay positive. I am pretty sure that if there is any child who can beat this disease it's Elena.

Day 9—DECEMBER 7

I guess you could call it regret—possibly remorse. But without a conclusion it doesn't quite feel like either. Today while waiting for a procedure with Elena, I saw a mother and a son sitting across from us. He was about eleven years old and was obviously a brain cancer patient. Although in very good spirits, he had undergone just about every surgery and procedure that you could imagine. He had lost his hair from aggressive chemotherapy, was undergoing his last MRI and radiation treatments and had a scar from the front of his brow to the back of his head with a shunt placed under the skin. Still, he had his personality and his sense of humor to go with the characteristic limp and facial paralysis that often come with brain surgery.

Was this what my daughter would have looked like if we had chosen the biopsy, the surgery and the chemotherapy? And even if we had this option with the type of tumor she has, could the outcome have been worse? I guess we'll never know, but the one question I can't avoid is whether our decision to treat this as a glioma rather than performing the biopsy cheats her of a complete cure. Sure, the odds are overwhelming and brain stem surgery almost never ends with a perfect conclusion. But then again, what are the odds of getting this type of tumor in the first place, in the worst possible place with one of the worst tumors out there? I guess, ultimately, it comes down to making the very best decision possible in enough time to prevent the inevitable complications that come with us exploring every option and doing every test. Still, these are questions that as a dad I will never escape.

Although she has had very few invasive procedures, Elena has had increasing difficulty with walking, talking and moving her right arm. For the first time I've also noticed that she can no longer make the kissing sound when she presses her lips up against my cheek. I'm going to miss that the most. At least her spirit is strong and her punch is as well. Right now she wants Mom more than Dad; after all, Dad teases and tickles while Mom cuddles and cares. And right now she needs more cuddling than teasing. Still, I manage to get a smile every now and then, about as much as I get a punch from her still strong left arm when she wants me to quit bothering her. That's when I tell her that if she wants to punch and kick me, she has to do it with her right side—the side that has the partial paralysis. I figure there's more than one way to approach therapy.

With the tumor progressing, her speech is now very limited and you can see her actively counting the amount of times she chews her food so she doesn't choke. I think she's as much aware of her situation as we are. Her tongue and palate paralysis are also making it very difficult to understand her words. She's getting visibly frustrated now and with her right hand almost completely immobilized, she has difficulty in helping convey her thoughts with hand motions. Brooke and I are now trying to teach her sign language in the event that she loses speech altogether, as well as her sight. Hopefully she will never have to use it, but we are painfully aware that this might be her only connection to the outside world. She already knows the alphabet A–E and knows the signs for "mother," "father," "thank you," "tree," "thirsty," "hungry" and "proud." We use the sign for "proud" the most throughout the day. Brooke is teaching her the sign for "bullshit" so at least she can curse when she gets frustrated. I don't think "shucks" has a sign. I keep telling her that as long as she keeps trying to tell us things, we'll keep working to understand; that way we'll never give up talking.

Day 10—DECEMBER 8

Today she got wheels. I guess we've known it was coming for the past week but chose to characterize it as the aftereffects of the anesthesia or exhaustion. Now we finally admit it is the tumor. There was no ignoring it when Elena woke up and her right hand was slightly bent with the fingers curled into her palm— the same way you often see in elderly patients with atrophy. She had the characteristic swelling of the right hand, the lint in the palm and the chapped fingers. We keep moisturizing her palm and trying to get her to move it, but it's no use. The therapist tells us that she will begin working with Elena next Tuesday, but that can't come soon enough; neither can the radiation.

In an effort to keep her hand active, we've started filling it with pudding cups and insisting that she feed herself. Actually, she insists on her independence as much as we do. Although not useful for many other things, her right hand is the perfect size to hold these cups and with her addiction to chocolate pudding, this comes in handy. Today alone she ate five pudding cups and three bowls of chocolate and vanilla swirl ice cream. Although we're trying to push vegetables, fruit and meat, with her swallowing issues we have a hard time getting her to eat them without choking.

Besides that, it's really tough to avoid spoiling her right now.

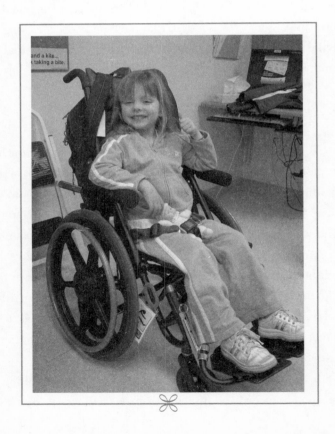

And we're not alone. With as many times as she has been in and out of the recovery room in the past week, the nursing staff has started to prepare swirl ice cream in advance of her procedures, just for her. For six years, Elena wanted nothing other than vanilla ice cream. Now all she wants is chocolate and vanilla swirl. Unfortunately, this is the one flavor they don't have. Still, that doesn't stop the nursing staff from mixing together a gallon of each flavor and freezing it in a special carton just for Elena. Now she has not only her own ice cream, but her own special shelf in the nurses' lunch freezer just for her.

Tonight Gracie arrived in Memphis with my parents and saw Elena at her worst. Hours after coming out of surgery and with steroids at an all-time high, she was in no mood for company, but a little Gracie time was exactly what she needed. Gracie has always been able to make Elena laugh, even in the worst of times. And today was one of those times. By the end of the evening they were laughing and fighting as usual. Gracie even had to try her hand at pushing Elena's wheelchair back and forth down the hallways until they both landed with a crash into the elevator wall. I think they both needed it, although Mom thought otherwise. Once again, Brooke was right and I was wrong.

Day 11—DECEMBER 9

For the past five years, we've never had a family portrait. It's not that we never had the time or the money but that we always figured that next year would be the year to do it. For a family of schedules, budgets and delayed gratification, it was never a priority—until now. This morning we finally had our picture taken—five years too late. We dressed up from the assortment of clothes we crammed into our bag just ten days before and forced smiles that we didn't feel inside. Then something happened—we rediscovered each other.

We discovered that Elena still had her infectious smile and model-like pose; Gracie was still the entertainer with her characteristic funny face and "antsy-pants" attention span. Mom was still the glue of the family with her beaming blue eyes and calming grace. I, on the other hand, was just the odd male out. And for twenty minutes we lived as we had two weeks ago, from picture to picture, and remembered a family that had it all because we had each other.

The experience was one I wish we had had every year. Oh how I wish I could look back upon the past years and say "Look at how young she was" or "She couldn't sit still then." Every picture tells a tale of the happier times—we just never took enough. And although the burdens of today will fade into what we will discover in the burdens of tomorrow, one thing will remain clear: the love expressed in those photos will help us overcome any challenge ahead. Take a picture.

Day 12—DECEMBER 10

Looking back, we're still glad we made the decision we made. Had we decided on a biopsy or surgery, radiation and chemotherapy wouldn't have started until after Christmas, which would have been too late. We've already noticed a decreased gag and choking reflex this morning, which would have surely meant a feeding tube procedure if we weren't going for radiation tomorrow. All the nurses and doctors tell us that she'll probably get worse before she gets better, but this will lessen as the tumor shrinks over the next couple of weeks. Whether her paralysis and speech will improve is yet to be seen, but we're already reminding her that the wheelchair is only temporary.

While she didn't want it in the first place, she now loves her new wheels. I think she likes getting pushed around all the time and getting all the attention she receives. But after one trip to the grocery store by myself, I can't wait to get rid of it. It's one thing to push a wheelchair, it's another to try pushing a shopping cart at the same time. After several attempts, we finally parked a cart at the end of the aisle and made trips back and forth. This worked until the third aisle, when someone took off with our cart and the food in it. At that point, I figured just the basics were enough and went for the bread and yogurt and called it quits. Enough for one day.

Day 14—DECEMBER 12

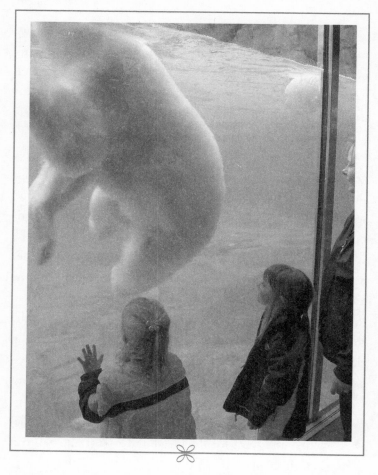

Her new nickname is Fred. At least that's what I call her when she tries to ignore the doctors and nurses. And it always gets a reaction. At first a slap with her remaining powerful left hand and then a smile begins to creep into her lips.

At first, I introduced her as "Fred George" when the bus

driver asked for her name and she responded by burying her face in her hand. I was not about to let her start out the day on a bad note.

From that point on, the name stuck. She was "Fred" to the receptionist, the nurses in radiation and just about anyone else who would listen. And by then, my little girl started to crack. The slaps became more forceful and so did the smiles. I knew it would only be a matter of time. The remainder of the day went wonderfully well; her attitude was positive, she didn't fear the radiation treatments quite as much (I'm being gracious with this; it still took its share of tears as she was sedated) and she actually began to speak in her speech therapy class. This alone was no small feat for a girl who had not uttered one word for the past four days. The words weren't clear or even loud, but it was an effort nonetheless.

Then, as quickly as it started, our day at the hospital was over. But no matter how much she wanted to rest, she had to see the animals. So off to the zoo we went. For the next forty minutes, the trip went something like this: "Oh, see the hippo. Oh, see the giraffe. Oh, see the lion. Oh, see the pengu—never mind, they're not out." Thirty seconds per animal doesn't afford you much time for reflection—especially with storm clouds looming overhead.

Then we saw the pandas, or shall I say P-A-N-D-A-S! Personally, I don't understand the lure of the panda. Why should they get their own house, their own velvet-rope lines and their own monuments, while the poor elephants get nothing more than a stinky house? Shouldn't the peacock at least get a small shrine? Apparently, I am in the minority and the rest of the world is in awe of the black-and-white-painted bears, including my daughter. For this we had to spend a good ten minutes admiring them, which meant we'd have to fast-walk the zebras, the gorilla and the antelope-looking thingies with the stripes (I think every zoo has thousands of these and no one knows what to call them) in order to catch up. Elena didn't care; these animals deserved a shrine in her mind as she pressed her nose up against the glass as close as she could without tipping over the wheelchair. And then came the smile. And then came the "Dad—take a picture" remark. And then she was Elena. I like pandas a little more now.

From there, we headed out the gates toward our car, but not before running into three Amish men visiting a patient at the hospital. Three hours earlier, they had walked to the zoo and now were second-guessing their decision as storm clouds loomed. So, in our infinite wisdom, we thought we'd corrupt the Amish men and offer them a ride back to the house in our car. Elena thought this was hilarious. I'm not sure if she understood the intricacies of this gesture, but she kept right on laughing anyway. And as we took off, one of the men joked, "I guess you've never driven the Amish," and Elena burst out laughing and continued all the way home. For the entire trip, she laughed elbow to elbow with three men in the backseat of the van. If there was ever a time for a picture, that would have been it. If only my camera battery would have allowed it. Oh well, that sort of thing happens every day. I'll get it next time.

Day 15—DECEMBER 13

Christmas is in full swing now at the hospital with donations coming in by the second and twenty or more toys for every patient. I think I have finally discovered the official Santa Claus imposter training camp, as we've had visits from over five Santas in the past four days. This doesn't do much for our whole Santa legend in Elena's eyes. I think she knows the truth, but she doesn't dare tell me. I think she thinks I still believe in him too and she doesn't want to spoil my Christmas.

Santa came again today. But by the fifth time, even Elena had reservations. With nothing left to do as we waited two hours for the next appointment, we decided to make the trip across campus. Apparently, we were not alone, as we entered a line of hundreds also waiting for a chance to see Santa. Within minutes, Elena was at the head of the line, herded into the 0–6 age group. There she was given a toy and a book that she immediately opened to read.

While a nice touch, this was unexpected—at least to us. From what we discovered, it was an annual event, as indicated by the crowd around us in the 0–6 line. Parents had not only known about it but had actively prepped their children for the event by instructing them to pick out the "most valuable" or the "in-demand" toy of the season from the selection. At that point, it ceased to be about what made the children happy and became more about what made the parents happy. There, all around me, were children who had been dragged out of beds from chemotherapy for the event just so they could claim a "prize" for the parents. And while some of these children chose to be there, there were also those who would rather have been in bed—anywhere but there. It almost seemed that the children were ashamed of their parents. I would be too. And not only had they planned for this event, but they also bragged to other families how they fooled a wish-granting organization into believing that their four-year-old wanted to go to Las Vegas as a last wish. I don't know about you, but I find it very hard to believe that any four-year-old chooses Las Vegas as his or her ideal vacation.

Was Elena thinking the same thing as I was? I don't know, but when it came time for her to choose, she chose the simplest $5 craft book on the table over a CD radio, a Disney Ariel musical instrument, an MP3 player and a Dora something-or-other in a giant box. With that, she asked to leave and motioned toward the door. I agreed. We left and sat on the grass reflecting on what we had just seen while we paged through the book.

Tragedy can both inspire and it can ruin lives. Some people use tragedy to exploit, and the ramifications of these actions hurt not only their own reputations, but the impressions of their children as well. Other people respond to tragedy with escapism and spoil their children. I'm as guilty as the next person. In the face of Elena's situation, I want to take her away from it all and show her the world. I want to skip the next six months of school and never let her out of my sight. I want to buy her that puppy I told her I was allergic to, that special toy that I never had enough money for and the prettiest clothes that don't come from a used clothes store. I want to give her everything. But in doing so, I know that I would also take away everything.

Normalcy is also a gift. She is homesick because she wants to go to school, because she wants her imperfect home, because she wants rules and discipline and because she wants her sister around. After all, in a way, our everyday lives are the lives we choose and hopefully the lives we've always wanted. This is the most that we can hope for: to be content with our lives and with ourselves. This is the gift I give my daughter and the gift I must keep giving her for the rest of her life, regardless of the length.

Elena wants to respect her family, wants to have her life back and doesn't want a toy or a trip in its place. In this way, her illness has taught us all a lesson in appreciation and giving thanks for what we already have. And although it may never be enough, it is what we need. We'll still take some vacations, we'll still treasure our time together, but from here on out, I will also honor her life as a five-year-old from Cincinnati with a foundation firmly rooted in traditions and morals. She'll have her family, her home, her school, her friends and her life back after radiation and chemotherapy treatments end two weeks from now. And if she wants a puppy after that, who knows, I may have to give up my allergy. Normalcy doesn't mean I won't always spoil her.

Day 16—DECEMBER 14

Over the past fifteen days, I've learned a few rules about medicine. First, a good bedside manner in pediatrics should never be underestimated. We've encountered fantastically prestigious doctors who knew nothing about Dora or Barbie and felt the solution to every problem was another IV line stuck into my daughter. We've also encountered doctors who freely admitted they were out of guesses but went out of their way to get to know Elena's birth date, that she preferred swirl ice cream over all others and that she would choose an Ariel sticker over a Jasmine sticker any day. And more often than not, it was the doctors with the good bedside manner who had the best results. Not because of what they knew, but because of what they discovered as Elena opened up to them. After all, in order to be a good investigator you have to uncover all the facts.

The second thing I've learned about medicine is that in order for it to work well, the patient needs to take an active role. The patient should not only understand the disease, but know when to direct the process if necessary. After all, it is your body or your child at stake. It will never be as high a priority to them as it is to you.

The third thing I've learned about medicine is that a good attitude and a positive outlook are critical to recovery. And while a disease may seem intimidating at first, there comes a time when you run out of tissues and you must work toward recovery. We're at this stage now.

The fourth thing I've learned about medicine is that strep throat causes brain tumors. Well, okay, maybe not, but it sure seems like it when you take your daughter to the hospital for a simple infection and you discover more than you ever wanted to know. I'm going for the MRI if Gracie ever gets a strep infection. Do you think it would be too much to just buy the machine and keep one in my basement just in case?

Seriously though, today was a day to say grace. Gracie Goose, specifically. And just as we discovered the importance of a positive outlook, Gracie came to save the day. You see, Elena and Gracie have never had anything in common other than their parents. Elena has brown hair; Gracie has blond hair. Elena has

Dad's nose (God help her) and Gracie has Mom's nose. Elena is the safe child, while Gracie is the one who will keep me up at night for the rest of my life (probably on the front porch with a shotgun in hand—you can never trust the boys). Elena has poise, and Gracie? Well, she has a sparkling smile and not one ounce of grace. (I told Brooke that she'd never have it if we named her Grace, but I'm never one to say I told you so.) Elena likes fancy nails and dresses; Gracie loves remote-control cars. Elena's serious and structured; Gracie is, well, Gracie. And she's just what Elena needs right now.

After spending a week hearing about tumors, radiation and hair loss, while struggling to keep down every bite of yogurt, Elena needed a dose of Gracie's spontaneity and unorthodox

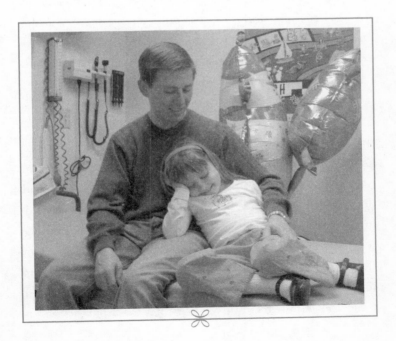

love. Of course, Grandma's love didn't hurt either. Thank goodness they arrived in Memphis just in time. And between the two of them they finally got Elena laughing and smiling within eight hours of their arrival. Before long, Elena was walking, talking, eating and smiling again. So what Dad and the doctors couldn't do in four days, Gracie and Grandma did in eight hours. And the recovery was miraculous. And while I'm sure the drug companies and the doctors will try to take credit for her improvement with the aid of radiation, dexamethasone, senna, ondansetron and whatever else she takes, Elena also got a prescription for love.

Grandma and Mom used their own prescription too. I'm sure the drug companies will immediately move to patent dress and shoe shopping when they discover the amount of improvement that Elena experienced after being led down the aisles of the local clothing stores in preparation for her big day at *The Nutcracker* on Saturday. It's amazing how much a red velvet dress and patent-leather red ballet shoes can do for cancer. Chances are it's probably cheaper than most of the drugs too.

Today was Gracie's big day and we all needed it. She has a way of stimulating excitement with her excessive energy and sparking smiles and with her simple yet perceptive comments. One minute she told me, "Geez, Dad, you know we wouldn't need all these doctors for Elena if we could just get Jesus to come down and fix her," and then the next minute she was explaining to me the difference between the Hello Kitty sticker that she wanted to give me and the Barbie sticker that she stuck to my shirt. She'd never repeat the comment, never discuss it, and for the life of me I don't know where these moments of brilliance come from, but with Gracie you know it comes from the heart at that very minute. Her passion is in the here and now, and Lord knows we need every bit of it we can get. And just in case you're curious, the difference between the Hello Kitty sticker and the Barbie sticker is that I'm not a girl so I must have more in common with a cat. Flashes of brilliance indeed.

Day 18—DECEMBER 16

It must be the ruby-red slippers. Elena wore them for the first time today and it made all the difference in the world. From morning till night, Elena walked nearly every hallway on her own power (of course with an overprotective Mom and Dad never leaving her side). Even when offered a ride on the wheelchair, she refused and kept right on going, struggling to lift the right leg against the strain of the paralysis and enduring atrophy. I think it was more a matter of will than a matter of strength today, as her spirits were high, her determination strong—and her fear of scuffing the shine of her brilliant new shoes. You see, Elena is one of those girls who prides herself on the shine of her shoes, so I knew that with every step she tried a bit harder to avoid dragging the right foot. Either way, it worked and I'll buy her new shoes every day if it continues to deliver progress.

The voice was improved today as she forced herself to use it, mostly directed at Gracie in screams of *"Mine,"* which were very clear indeed. The rest of the words and sentences were still mostly unclear, but the important part was that she tried. After all, therapy is more a struggle of determination than it is a matter of ability. Hopefully this will continue to improve over the next couple of days as Mom takes over.

And this is where I started eighteen days ago with a diagnosis and an unfamiliar new world. For the first time, I will leave Elena's side to head back to Cincinnati while Mom takes over for the next four days. Since we learned of the tumor eighteen days ago I've spent every night and every day by Elena's side. We've had conversations about lifetime wishes and arguments about Muppets, both with an intensity that I never before thought possible. She's a fan of Rizzo, while I'm partial to Gonzo. The rift could never be greater. At the same time, I learned more about my daughter in eighteen days than I'd learned about her in five years, eleven months and twenty-six days. She likes painting more than drawing, prefers nightgowns without sleeves and loves chocolate/vanilla swirl ice cream over everything else. If they don't have that, she'll take plain vanilla, but never chocolate ice cream alone. And in that time, I watched her progress from a limp and a weak voice to right-side paralysis, limited left-side vision and no voice at all. Now she has come full circle back to where we started with a right-side limp and a weak voice. Physically, it is like the last eighteen days never happened, but in our minds we know better. At points, I even wondered if we would make it this far as we encountered internal-bleeding scares, choking and a tumor that seemed to outrun the most aggressive steroid treatments that were prescribed. While not something I wish to repeat, this time solidified our priorities and made us ready for the struggle ahead.

Today was also a day that taught us to embrace that struggle as we took Elena out on the town. First, she went with Mom, Gracie and my mother for a manicure, pedicure and hairstyle. It was a chance to be pampered by the folks at the local beauty school and a moment to take pride in how she looked. And although the moment was fleeting due to the pain she experienced from the medicine she took that morning, it was enough to change her frame of mind and dissolve the glum look she had carried throughout the week. Once again she felt like a little girl as she showed off her fingernails and toenails to anyone who would stop to look. With a special trip to *The Nutcracker* tonight, the red nails and shoes to match were critical.

The Nutcracker has been a wish of Elena's for some time now, ever since she first saw the nutcrackers that we displayed on the fireplace mantel last year. And after Brooke explained the significance and the ballet connection, Elena was mystified. So when the first tree went up at the local hardware store after Halloween (hey, it's the store that I take her to the most), she knew it was time for the *Nutcracker* play. Now she would finally get to go to her first ballet in a real theater with a fancy dress, pretty nails and a hairstyle. And she was in heaven. Of course, she also wore the ruby-red slippers to complete the outfit.

I'd love to say she was in awe of every minute or that she idolized every ballerina, but the truth is that she fell asleep after intermission in Mom's arms. Radiation takes its toll on a child in terms of exhaustion and this was its effect. But the impact was still there. It was an afternoon away from the anesthesia, the chemotherapy and the blood tests—and that's what mattered most. It was also a chance to cuddle in Mom's arms and I'm sure that was fine with Mom as well. Gracie, on the other hand, was a bundle of energy as she bounced between Grandma's lap and mine, mimicking the arm motions of every last soldier, snowflake princess and sugarplum fairy onstage. Occasionally, she would grow tired of this as well and would resort to rubbing Grandpa's beard and hair for good luck, kissing his cheek.

All in all, it was a good day. And the satisfaction I have in leaving tomorrow morning after seeing this improvement will be offset by the realization that according to the doctors, this progress might very well be temporary. It's always hard to see your

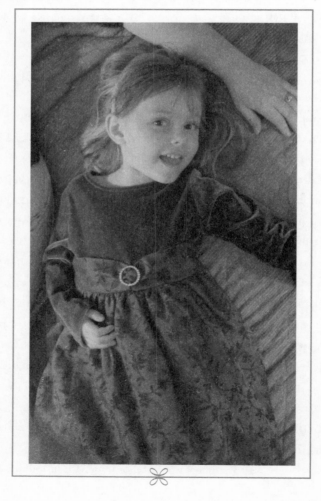

once healthy daughter reduced to paralysis, an arsenal of drug treatments and a possible terminal illness all in a matter of days. I imagine it is much harder to see her improve to her previous perfection only to wonder how long it will last. Will it be three months, five months, seven months or possibly the rest of her life? She is definitely improving and from what I can see, she might regain all previously lost abilities. Our biggest fear is that after she improves she might quickly regress. For this reason, Brooke and I focus on her treatments, possible cures and learning sign language as a method of communication if she were to lose her eyesight and ability to talk when the tumor returns again one day.

Of course, we will always pray for a miracle, but the reality is that we must also prepare for the inevitable. At the same time, we realize the lesson to be learned in terms of life's priorities and focusing on family above everything else. It has been eighteen days and we have our Elena back. It has been eighteen days and we now know her better than ever. And with these eighteen days in mind, we have also discovered a determination and will in our daughter that we never saw before. If this is any indication of her strength, I doubt we will ever need those sign language classes.

Day 22—DECEMBER 20

Tomorrow is Elena's sixth birthday. Somehow we never imagined spending it this way. While other children anticipate a big cake, a new bike or weeklong celebrations, we want nothing more than time. And yet it's the one present that I can't buy.

Six years ago, Elena taught me to be a father. Once brash and selfish, I was quickly humbled by the delicate touch of her hand wrapped around my fingers. Born at a little over five pounds, she quietly snuggled in the warmth of my forearm, preemie clothes ill fitting and draped over her tiny body. Without a tear or a cry even as a baby, she taught us how to be better parents and had patience that seemed unusual for her age. Even in the middle of the night, I'd awake to her cooing rather than crying and understand what she wanted. And there we'd spend the early morning hours, asleep in the chair beside her crib, waiting for the alarm in the next room to start the new day.

Life had new meaning and every action had a purpose. I began to see the world from the eyes of a father. Working was about feeding my family, the nightly news suddenly became worrisome and education became a priority. Still, each night was

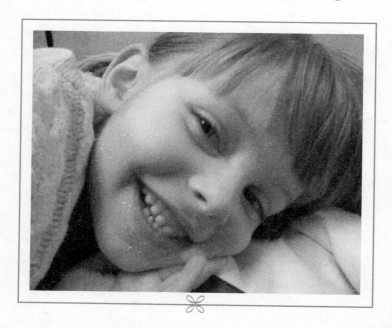

about Elena and the concerns of the day, and fatherhood would have to wait. And from her very first week until her sixth year, we'd sit peacefully on the porch or deck ending the day with each other. As a baby she'd lie in my arms, but as she grew older she'd sit by my side, her toes brushing the grass below. And in every way she was my equal and hero. Today it is no different.

In six years we've learned a great deal about Elena. Once a baby, she is now a little girl, brimming with personality and charm. But instead of planning her future, we now find ourselves counting days. Somehow I can't imagine a worse diagnosis or a worse time to lose her. So we hope, pray and remember. It's all that we can do while we count days and tell her that everything will be all right. I just hope it is.

Day 23—DECEMBER 21

Six years—and yet the days seem to move faster than ever now. It is Elena's sixth birthday today and she started it out with a frown and a bit of 'roid rage. Not even the bus driver could coax a smile out of her on the lift ride into the bus. But her mood soon changed as we exited radiation recovery by noon and went to the cafeteria for lunch. There she had what she called a "small" breakfast of cheese eggs, yogurt, a bowl of oatmeal and milk. Looked bigger to us. Then, no more than one hour later, she wondered what was for lunch.

From there, we went back to the hospital for a schedule and to hand out gifts to our angels of the brain tumor ward. Elena gave out her handwritten cards from her private stash and a bit of "bling" to the women in the form of a Christmas tree pin that she had picked out earlier that weekend. For the men she had a nutcracker in mind. She seems to have taken to the entire nutcracker theme as of late. She sleeps with a nutcracker at the head of her bed and insists that we put them on the mantel at home. This is her decoration and her mark on Christmas. I'm not sure of the symbolism, but it's her new Christmas tradition.

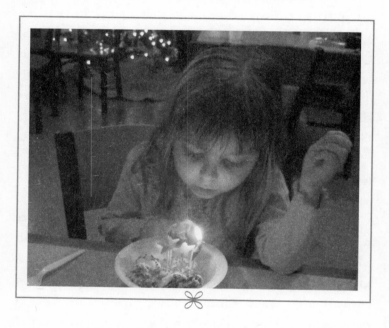

The staff of the brain cancer ward had their own party in mind: Elena's nurse headed up a birthday committee in Elena's honor. And there with the confetti that they had so eagerly manufactured from hole-punching just about every piece of colored paper in the office earlier, they sang "Happy Birthday" to Elena and lightened our load with a flock of balloons large enough to start a voyage around the world. As we went from appointment to appointment, we spread the joy, dragging confetti from clinic to clinic as it rubbed off of our clothes and hair and fell from the wheelchair. I have no doubt that the janitor will easily be able to determine our schedule for the day. And with the balloons attached to every bar on the wheelchair, we completed the day and headed back to the room—but not before running into every wall, corner and person that we failed to see through the screen of balloons.

Tonight, Elena fell asleep smiling. Her voice has improved, she can now eat some real food, her right arm is starting to work again and she now walks around the room by herself. All is good and improving—thank God. Happy birthday, Elena!

Day 24—DECEMBER 22

Time is precious. I learned this being away from Elena for the past three days. And when I returned to Memphis on Wednesday evening, I breathed a sigh of relief. Just as Keith had discovered the previous week, when I went back to Cincinnati to work, I spent every minute thinking of Elena and wanting to be back in Memphis. And I mean every minute. You see, when I went back to Cincinnati I couldn't sleep. It wasn't because I wasn't tired or because I was just that busy, it was because I now see sleep as a waste of time. It's amazing how an experience such as this changes your philosophy on life. And while we never really slept in—6 A.M. was "sleeping in" for us, even on the weekends— every minute that you spend away from your daughter with a critical illness is a minute that you lose. So what do you do? You clean the house, rearrange her room, put up Christmas decorations and write in a journal until 2 in the morning. And the most surprising thing is that we're not tired—this is just the new norm.

The same thing applies to the holiday spirit. Today, while waiting for the bus, Keith and I wondered what we'd be doing now had Elena not developed cancer. We'd probably be running around town looking for that last-minute gift, swearing to ourselves as we stood in line, waiting in traffic and working until 7 o'clock at night. We'd complain that we didn't have enough time or money or the perfect holiday decorations. Now there's so much more to consider but less to worry about. We look back at pictures from Halloween and think to ourselves how naïve and lucky we were, but we never really knew it at the time. It's funny how you never know how much you can handle until it gets worse. And just when you get used to that, it happens again. But somehow, even with this experience you find a way to make it work because that is how you cope. Not because you deserve it or because you need the experience to set priorities, but because it's the human thing and it is life. And through this experience we will grow, find out what the holiday means and learn to expect more of each other. Together we will use this struggle to make us stronger as a family and support each other when we break down. That is what a family does and how we cope.

Day 25—DECEMBER 23

Today was a day of hope. It was also the day of Elena's birthday party—two days late. But after driving through the night, we were glad to be back home. Originally we planned on having Elena's birthday party at the local gymnastics romper room like just about every other suburban family, but in light of her condition and her wishes, we opted for the local chili parlor up the street to allow for her friends to visit. I think she enjoyed this best. So putting on her second-best dress (sorry to all at the party, but the best dress is for Christmas), she left with Mom for a morning at the spa, where she had her nails polished and her hair curled.

And while I'm not sure that anyone has ever gone to the spa and dressed in their best clothes to go to a chili parlor, it is what made Elena happy and that's all that mattered.

On arrival, Elena shunned her wheelchair as she decided that today was the day to try her new leg brace. After all, what good are fancy clothes if you have to sit in them all day? But when she resisted holding our hands for balance, we finally understood her motives and resorted to corralling her on both sides with our hands in case she fell. She didn't.

Somehow, the folks at the restaurant had gotten the impression that we had a party of fifty or less, but within half an hour we filled up the party room and had started to conquer the rest of the restaurant as well. And by the end of the party, close to eighty people had come to visit Elena on her first trip home. Family, friends, schoolteachers, coworkers (she comes to work with Mom and me in the morning and they consider her the "real" boss), more family and even people we never met before joined us in celebrating her birthday. Even her friends from her kindergarten class came. For the past week, these were the ones I heard about as she planned her visit home. Now I saw the joy on her face as she hugged each one, wishing she too could be outside on the school playground every morning, freezing while waiting for the bell, as I imagine they must be doing this time of year. It was truly a day to remember even if it was nothing more than hot dogs and cheese.

Tonight Brooke cried. But unlike before, it wasn't because of anticipation or grief, but because she saw how many people truly cared. These are the tears we need more of every day to ensure that Elena wins her fight.

Day 26—DECEMBER 24

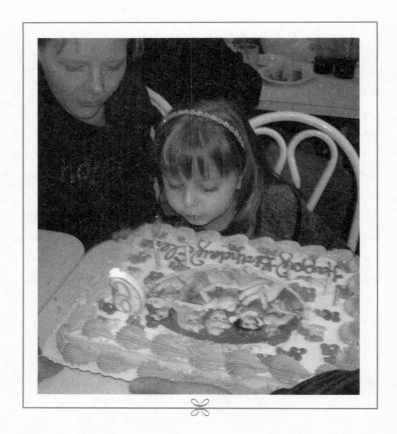

When you take care of Elena, you're focused on the present. What dosage of steroids is the right dose? What are the side effects of chemotherapy? Can she handle the leg brace instead of the wheelchair? And each of these pursuits focuses your efforts on beating the disease one step at a time. At first you resent the monotony of the schedule as opposed to a quick and fast solution. Then, as you realize the scope of childhood cancer, it soon becomes a crutch as you can see daily improvement that forces you to believe Elena will win. Sometimes this improvement doesn't come and sometimes you see regression, but in the long run you see your daughter change and develop. One step at a time the depression will erode. The isolation and the fear, however, are always present.

In Cincinnati you are forced daily to come to terms with the future. This is probably the most painful part of it all. Here you drive past the school every morning and wonder if you'll get to help with Halloween snacks with Elena in first grade, if Gracie and she will appreciate sharing a bathroom when they're teenagers and how you'll teach her to drive a stick shift. Here reside the questions of the unknown that make it especially hard to continue daily activities. In time, this too will pass as she improves and we learn to live in Cincinnati day-to-day just as we do in Memphis. Perhaps this will happen as soon as February, when she returns to Cincinnati and we can begin to live life again—but not in the same way.

For the next month, this will be our life. One day at a time.

Day 27—DECEMBER 25

Our Christmas gift was Elena this year. At 3:30 in the morning she woke us up at home to the sound of her voice when she came in to tell us that she wanted to watch cartoons. Her voice was clear and not nasal, as it had been since Thanksgiving. And despite both of us being sound asleep, Brooke and I shot out of bed in amazement. A small piece of us wondered if it had all been just a bad dream and our daughter was fine after all. Then reality set in as she explained that her voice felt better and she had taken a drink of water and it helped her voice. And at 3:30 in the morning, we carried on a conversation. Her voice only lasted for a short time, but we ignored our bloodshot eyes and carried on the conversation—never mind that this was the first night that we could have slept more than four hours consecutively. How sweet the sound!

Christmas also brought many more gifts in the form of her continued walking, her eating nuts, fruits and pizza, and the first time she joined Gracie for tickle time on the floor of the family room. But most of all, what I'll remember about this Christmas is making her smile.

At first it wasn't easy. When we dragged her out to church and then to my aunt's Christmas celebration, she refused to participate and sat grudgingly with her head in her hands. No toy, person or visit from Santa could change her outlook. And although a visit from Sally (my aunt's ten-inch-tall Chihuahua with a case of the shakes and beady eyes) induced a smile, it quickly faded as the never-ending hunger pains set in for the fourth time in less than an hour. Food drive and the power of steroids!

No, above all, it was the things that she refused to do that gave her the most joy. You see, Elena never does anything of her own will. If you ask her to water-ski, she refuses and says, "Maybe tomorrow." If you ask her to read her reading primer she says, "I can't right now." If you ask her to try her bike without training wheels you get "I'm too young." That's where Gracie comes in. Gracie will do anything, anytime, regardless of whether she can do it right or whether she will get hurt. "Act first, think later" is Gracie's motto. Her other motto is "I'm all right," when she picks herself up off the ground after falling. And while I cringe at the thought of her as a teenager, I love having her attitude right now.

When Elena says, "Maybe tomorrow," I simply turn to Gracie, who always accepts. Not even a second passes before Elena reconsiders and turns competitive. Before long, she's water-skiing, riding that bicycle and sounding out every word. Now of course, Gracie can't ride that bike (balance is not her virtue), and Gracie can't read yet (although she's getting pretty close). But when I hold the back of the bike so it looks like she's doing it herself and when I act like Gracie is whispering the words in my ear, Elena immediately has to do one better. Sometimes I think Elena teaches Gracie caution, while Gracie teaches Elena courage. It's a great combination.

This time, it was driving. Yes, driving. You see, we had about thirty minutes to kill before church and I thought it would be a good idea to teach Elena how to drive. After all, I only have another ten years to teach her so I better get started. Mom, on the other hand, didn't agree. "What are you, stupid?" she asked. I too can be competitive, so off I went with my little stunt. After asking Elena and being turned down, I went to Gracie. All I needed to do was look at Gracie and she was immediately in my lap, ready to go. And for the next ten minutes, Captain Zigzag was at the helm as we drove from one edge of the parking lot to the next and occasionally almost into a post or two. She loved it as she donned my sunglasses to get the complete effect.

Elena had to be next. She was labeled the Queen of the Grass as we took off through the abutting field and over a curb or two. She loved it. And for the next fifteen minutes she squealed, laughed and giggled. I think we'll have to do it again. Maybe tomorrow.

For most kids, gifts at Christmas would have been the most

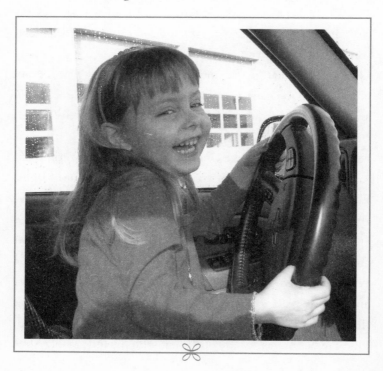

important part of the holiday. For Elena, this Christmas was different. And while she opened the gifts, most were left by the edge of the tree as she moved on to the next. Instead, Elena got more joy out of giving me my gift than any of the ones she received. Apparently, she and Mom went shopping together and decided that I needed a balloon animal kit. So for the next two hours, Christmas stopped while Elena and I sat next to each other laughing. I'm not ready for the restaurant circuit, but I do have a pretty good assortment of animals to choose from. I can make snakes, giraffes with short legs, dogs with long necks, horses with long necks and short legs, and even butterflies without wings that look like long-necked dogs. Not bad if I do say so myself. And it only takes two balloons to get one that doesn't pop. That's skill. Elena thinks I should make balloons for the doctors at the hospital tomorrow. I promise to as long as she promises to try the radiation without sedation. What she doesn't know is that I'll do it for nothing more than a smile. What a deal.

Day 28—DECEMBER 26

She certainly didn't want to be back at the hospital. Neither did I after driving through the night to get back to Memphis. Just getting her out of bed at 5 A.M. proved impossible as she clung to her pillow, squeezing out every last bit of sleep. And this was the same girl who came to our bedside every morning at 3 on weekends. The same medicine regimen that took no more than ten minutes over the weekend now took thirty minutes, as she first refused the Jell-O that contained the pill and then spit out the pill rather than swallow it.

The radiation treatments came later that day. This too was difficult as I tried to continue the work that Brooke had started last week with getting her to stay still during the radiation treatments while awake. Up until now, Elena has needed sedation in order to remain still during her radiation treatments. And this means she has to take the "white medicine" that not only sedates her but also makes her very nauseous. Our first experience with this nausea came a few minutes into the IMAX movie at the local museum of natural history, where I took Elena to change the mood a bit. Elena began to complain of stomach pain, and without a bathroom in sight, I ended up using the only other thing I had—my hands. Eventually, this translated into my shirt, her shirt and her pants until we finally found the bathroom and attempted to clean up.

And there, in the men's bathroom, as she stood in her underwear while I dressed her in the only change of clothes I had (an old diaper bag from Gracie's baby years was in my car with two-year-old summer clothing), she asked *the* question. "Why does this have to happen to me?"

Not thinking much of the question, I answered that it happens to a lot of kids in the theater and it can also happen to most children who are getting radiation. Not satisfied with the answer, she touched my head and asked again, "No, Dad, why am I sick with the bump in my head when all of my friends are not?"

I had been asking the same question for a month. And somehow the answer never fits since it should never happen to any child in the first place. To simply pass it off as "odds" is to say that you'd be fine if it was someone else's child. To tag it as a "message from God" is to create a doubt of faith if you are the one who loses your child to the "message." In the end, I don't think you ever have an answer because there are no right answers. It happens and you learn to deal with it, fight it or accept it—all very different responses by different people.

Now I'd love to tell you that I came up with a cute answer that tied it all together. And for the purposes of this journal, I'd like to at least find some meaning, but I have none. The truth is that I looked at my daughter, shrugged and said, "It will be all right," and hugged her. That's it. Someday, I hope to answer that question and in doing so, improve her life, mine and a thousand others', but for now I'm forced to be humble and give her the reassurance she desperately needs. That's the mission of a father: to reassure and protect.

Day 29—DECEMBER 27

She can roll her tongue! I know it doesn't seem like a big deal to most people, but to me it is everything. You see, one of the first things that she lost when the tumor took over was the ability to roll her tongue. Then she lost her voice, her right hand, her right leg, her peripheral vision and her ability to swallow. So to get the tongue back is a very big deal. Sure, the leg is still a bit slow, but what this means to me is that we're getting everything back and Elena is getting better. Hopefully it will all stay that way. I know every day from here on out will begin with me asking her to roll her tongue as she crawls out of bed. Who needs MRI and CT equipment when all you need is a roll of the tongue?

Day 31—DECEMBER 29

All around us I see examples of determination, love and commitment to living. They are the children age twelve and up, those who have been here before. They have experienced relapses, possibly for the second, third or even fourth time. And their wisdom and resolve are what drive us each and every day.

Today I sat on a bus with Elena as we traveled back to the house. In a nearby seat sat a father and a daughter. They too are heroes. He sat along the aisle, she sat next to the window—just as Elena and I sat behind them. She was about five years older than Elena and had been here before. Her father sat nearby, looking for conversation to break the thoughts of the nausea that his daughter undoubtedly felt. During the five-minute drive, barely a word was spoken between them, but I knew they did not need small talk to communicate. When we arrived, he rose and helped her to her feet, and she stepped forward determined to leave the bus on her own power. I looked at Elena and saw her in five years. I wondered if we too would return, or would we experience a miracle and never return? Would she be a hero as well? And while I never want to see Elena go through a relapse, I realize that in her case the miracle might be just making it five years.

Elena is doing well today and I hope she will continue to improve over the coming months. Of course, we will have complications and side effects, but regardless of the struggle, I pray we will succeed. I know she will be a hero. She already is.

Day 32—DECEMBER 30

I look out the window and have thoughts I should never have. I look back at my daughter lying in bed and compare what I see. Outside the hospital I see drug deals, prostitution and wasted opportunities. Inside our room I see a little girl fighting for her life. Outside, they have all the time in the world, while inside, Elena's life might be reduced to days and hours. It isn't fair. I guess I shouldn't expect it to be.

It goes on twenty-four hours a day. On the streets outside the hospital, the comparisons are obvious. I am frustrated and angry. But then again it doesn't make sense. Isn't her life more precious? As I said, these are questions I should never ask.

We all waste our time and our lives when we should aspire to do more. What we all wouldn't do for just one more day when it comes to an end. The loss of a child represents every lesson we should learn and every moment we should cherish. But instead, we follow the foolish, ignore the clock and cry victim when consequences fall. Yet these children get no such warning. Elena was never foolish, never ignored the clock, and she is in a battle for her life. She becomes a lesson for us all. My price may be my daughter.

I will never understand and that's the irony of it all. The ultimate lesson here is one that I will never agree with or ever hope to find inspiration in. I don't fight to help other children because of Elena's lesson; I fight to help other children because I don't want the lessons to continue. I love my daughter and no lesson is worth her life. I will continue even if she loses her fight.

I will always remember these nights in the hospital as she slept softly and I sat by her side, peering into the darkness outside. It wasn't fair. Nothing is worth taking the life of a child. It doesn't make sense—but then again, it's not supposed to.

Day 34—JANUARY 1

This morning started in a flurry of activity. After an eight-hour drive back home, everyone slept in today. Then the girls came into our bedroom and we all slept in a little more. I remember just six months ago groaning when the girls woke us up early on the weekends and promptly ushering them upstairs to watch cartoons while we caught a few more minutes of sleep. Now we don't mind the wake-up call and snuggle up with them even longer. Too bad we're only home for a day and then back to Memphis.

Day 36—JANUARY 3

I was approached twice today by fellow mothers remarking on how Elena has made such a wonderful recovery. I am torn. On one hand, I smile and think to myself that it truly is a miracle that these changes have occurred in two weeks. On the other hand, I hate to get too comfortable with the recovery. I keep finding myself forgetting that this may be temporary. I find myself slipping back into old habits of working when we get home rather than playing with her, reading a newspaper rather than squeezing every last ounce of conversation out of her, thinking about everything I left undone at home rather than what things I haven't done with Elena.

Those who know me best know I don't like surprises. I am a "read the last chapter of a book first" kind of girl. I need to know what is ahead of me so I can plan out each step to get there. I find myself in a weird sort of depression. I know what the future holds (or the most probable one) but I am paralyzed. I sit across from this little girl every day, cracking jokes and learning subtraction, and I have a horrible thought. These treatments have done wonderful things and fixed all the problems this tumor has caused, but did they make her too normal? I look at Elena and have a really hard time imagining that we could have a recurrence. Most look at that and say this is a good thing and positive thinking is the best course of action. I am scared that we will get too comfortable and this stupid tumor is going to broadside us. So do you live with the knowledge that it will grow again and try to cram a lifetime into a year? Or do you live with a positive outlook and maintain the status quo?

Aside from her ever-growing cheeks and healthy appetite, Elena is back to normal. It must be very weird for her to feel back to normal and still be stuck in a hospital. Actually, going home for the holidays helped her so much. She can now visualize herself getting better, going to school, playing with her sister and most important, being the "Razzle Dazzle" girl of the week in her kindergarten class.

Day 42—JANUARY 9

Tonight Elena wants to write in the journal. Here goes—I'll help spell:

Hi, everybody!

I can't wait to come home.

My favorite animal is a hummingbird but I don't have a feeder
for one yet.

I like to wear skirts and sparkly headbands.

I like to read my animal book with all the animals inside.

I like to watch cartoons when I get back from the hospital.

> My favorite show is <u>Go, Diego, Go!</u> because it's all about a
> rescue and Diego really likes animals like me.

My most favorite thing to do with my Gracie is to play outside.

My favorite color is pink.

My most favorite part about school is eating lunch and being
Razzle Dazzle.

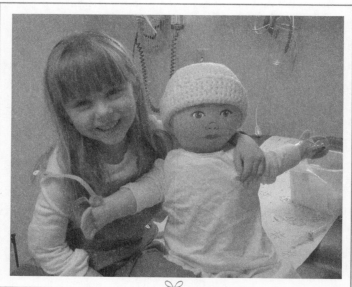

My favorite season is summer because you get to go to the
  beach.
Soccer is my favorite sport.
The first thing I want to do when I get home is go to the beach.
The one thing I wish I could do is swim with fish.
The least favorite thing about the hospital is the needle in my port.
I loved when everyone sang to me for my birthday.

Day 45—JANUARY 12

"You don't know me but . . ." It's the way most of the cards
sent to Elena begin. And what started as an innocent journal for
Gracie about her sister has now become so much more. Our daily
journal started as a remembrance as we first came to grips with
her illness, but it has now become the driving force in her recovery. Every day brings more cards, more letters and more e-mails
than we can possibly read to her. Every day we pack cards for
the hospital waiting room and pass the time reading to her the
greetings from friends and family. It brings a smile to her and it
brings encouragement to us. And now, for the first time, I can
see the positive once again with the blessings of Elena's friends.

The cards come from all over: Ohio, Kentucky, Indiana,
Iowa, Pennsylvania, Florida, Tennessee, Georgia, Alabama,
New York, California, Washington, Maryland, Virginia, Michi-
gan, Texas, Illinois, Arizona, Arkansas and plenty of other states
I don't even remember at this time. Each one offers get-well
wishes, birthday greetings and holiday cheer. Some carry pho-
tographs, some carry children's drawings and some carry small
gifts, but all deliver smiles.

The cards now cover her door, obscure her bulletin boards and hang from the ceiling of her bedroom. Each of them carries a message—a message of hope. Hope for her health, hope for her happiness, hope for her future. For us, they carry us through every day.

Day 47—JANUARY 14

Do you ever know when you are experiencing a miracle? I guess I just expected more—maybe a flash of light, a clap of thunder or a visit from an angel. But maybe, just maybe, the angel is right here next to me.

It's true that Elena has come so far so fast. Of course, she also lost so much so quickly. But now she's back—smiles and all. And as I watch her run from swing to swing with her Pippi Longstocking tights, I truly begin to appreciate what we once had—all over again.

Today was a day to relax. Unfortunately it was already too short. In an effort to get away from the hospital, we decided to visit my sister in Alabama. Mom and Gracie left and, after a picnic in the park, so did Grandma and Grandpa. Then it was back to Aunt Jackie's house to relax and spend a couple of hours driving in the same loop around the backyard in the mini Jeep (boy does she love that thing). But after the fourth battery charge only lasted twenty minutes, Elena knew it was time to settle down with her cousins.

While the agenda was light, the memories were powerful. And somehow, some way, if I try hard enough, the day will never end. How do you know if a miracle is happening? You don't, but as a parent I'd just love to experience the peace of knowing that I'll get to see her graduation, her wedding and her children. But for now, you focus on the many miracles that occur every day. Sixty miracles in a minute; 3,600 in an hour; 86,400 in a day—one miracle per second.

Day 48—JANUARY 15

"Free at last . . . free at last!" I think Elena has listened to a bit too much CNN on Martin Luther King Jr. Day. Although certainly appropriate considering her improvement, I never figured I'd hear her singing this as she rode around Aunt Jackie's yard in circles on the mini Jeep. Too bad we had to leave it all behind and travel back to Memphis.

Free at last, most certainly. With only ten days left before we leave the hospital and return home, Elena has become the elder stateswoman of the house. She knows the routine, knows her fellow patients and knows the staff. Upon arriving back at the house, she informed me that we were to eat dinner (the cheese pizza in the freezer was her choice), then check mail and finally finish back at the room with a pint of ice cream and a Muppet movie. And although her head never crested the front counter as she asked for the mail and she couldn't get the security code to work when we made our way to the front door, it was clear that she was in charge. She chose the meal, she helped make it and she set the table. I figure she feels that either I'm in over my head kitchen and get the Oreos from the pantry. After all, she claimed Mom did this every night. Aha!! And all that talk about being good—now I understand how Mom made it through two weeks at the house.

Elena has improved greatly over the past weeks, but her walking and her balance are still missing. I was reminded of this as we approached the stairway to our second-floor room. With a tug at my side, she again needed my help to climb the steps. I guess I could have taken the elevator, but without steps I would never get the opportunity to carry her and get free kisses. You see, every three steps require a kiss from Elena in order to continue. It's like Daddy fuel. And the way I figure it, with twenty-four steps total to the top, I get at least eight kisses every time. Of course, I usually fake a step just to get nine kisses. I think she knows, but she gives it to me anyway. As independent as Elena is getting, I can use all the opportunities I can get. Who needs Oreos when you get this?

Day 49—JANUARY 16

I remember when Elena was intimidated by school. First, she was scared of day care. Then she was scared of the first day of kindergarten. She wrapped her little arms around Mom's legs and shed the customary tears. Day two brought even more tears. I guess when you know what to expect, it can be even more fearful. Day three through day seven saw fewer tears, bashful hel-
los to teachers and friends

took at least five kisses and hugs before she would leave our side, but looking back I wish it would have taken at least six or more.

Yes, we were the "left-over parents," the ones who still walked our children to the door when everyone else sought the protection of their warm cars when the cold temperatures came home to roost. Sure, there were a few more additions after weekends and absences, but we were the "regulars" of the group. To this day, I don't know if it was because she needed the support or whether we couldn't let go, but it doesn't matter now. I'll be there every morning from now until she goes to college, maybe even longer. Sure, it's a little protective, but think of how much she'll appreciate it when she goes to high school and I'm walking five feet behind. She can look over her shoulder, introduce me to her friends and thank me for accompanying her. Okay . . . maybe not.

What was different about Elena was not how she entered school but how she left. When most kids left screaming out the door, relieved to be finished, Elena would talk about how much she missed it from the moment she walked out the door. She'd tell me about art, about share-chair, about lunch, and she'd tell me about her plans for tomorrow. Even on the weekends she'd play teacher, complete with her pointer and blackboard. This was the role Elena was born to play. Poor Gracie; she did nothing other than raise her hand for the last four years.

When Elena came to the hospital and was subjected to a seemingly endless barrage of tests and drugs, you could easily understand her depression. Everyone was treating the body and no one was treating the mind. No creativity, no learning, no advancement. While her body recovered, her mind was at a point of atrophy. They offered psychological sessions, movie nights and even gifts, but none had any effect. So when we discovered the educational center at the hospital, we quickly knew the answer.

I've figured out that kids just aren't that complex. We think they need understanding and comforting when all they really need is a challenge and a bit of truth. A month ago, Elena craved both. She knew she had something very bad; why else would she get all this attention? So after two months of hiding our meetings behind locked doctors' doors, she made us discuss it in front of her. And in a way, it forced us to reconcile with the positives as well as the negatives of the disease. As for a challenge, she only had to be provided with the opportunity to learn and she was determined to take it from there. School was that answer, and today we found out that the hospital provides schooling in the lower-level basement.

As a result, her attitude is better than it has ever been before. She's not only happy with herself, but probably more confident now than she was at home. And while she still hangs on to my legs at every doctor visit, she never forgets when it is time for school. It is the first question she asks when I get the schedule for the next day and I'm amazed at her grasp of time when she reminds me about her "school appointment" within minutes of its start. Then, without asking, she's off to the elevator and on her way to class. With her rolling backpack, she pushes past nurses and patients, leaving me to follow. God help me if I get distracted—I know she'll never wait.

School is a purpose and a routine. It is what she loves about her life and what she needs right now to be a child again. It's not just about education anymore.

Day 50—JANUARY 17

Congratulations! You have cancer.

I look around the hospital and see the signs of friends and family trying to cope with the news. The child who was healthy yesterday is terminal today. And we do the best we can to help.

Sadly there are few options and very little we actually can do. In Elena's case there may be none. So we give her toys, buy her clothes and spoil her.

At the hospital it's no different. And in every room the toys lay unopened in the corner waiting to be replaced by the next visitor bearing gifts. Elena's closet is packed with new clothes, fancy hats and the most glorious collection of tights that her grandmother can buy. Yet most of the tags remain intact. There will never be enough time to wear everything or play with every toy. Even Elena knows this and has stopped opening the gifts.

It's not that she doesn't appreciate the gesture. She smiles and gives out hugs. It's just that she wants something more; she wants to be normal. She wants to be healthy. But that is the one gift that can't be wrapped.

We try our best to understand, but we don't and never will. They ask her what she wants to do as a "wish trip." She shrugs and doesn't answer. I tell the volunteer she wants to be healthy. Elena listens, hoping that there's a chance. It's the volunteer's turn to shrug. She doesn't have an answer for this. So we take a brochure and go back to the room to rest and prepare ourselves for the next day.

Cures don't come on toy shelves and they don't have tags. And while we have all the toys a little girl could ever desire, faith now comes in short supply. So we do what we can: we spoil them, treat them like princesses and buy everything they ever wanted. And in a way, it's like a prize for getting cancer. Suddenly we care, suddenly we love and suddenly we buy them the world. But it's too late. All she wants now is to be normal.

Day 51—JANUARY 18

At the hospital boardinghouse you start as unknowns, only to become family. With its common kitchens, family rooms and support programs, you soon share experiences, memories and concerns with the other fifty families. When Elena and I first arrived, we were strangers, having moved to the house one week prior to the rest of the families at the hospital. While we were settling in, most of the other families were moving out. But then our generation started to arrive and one by one we began to understand their plights as well.

Five weeks later, everything changes. With most families nearing their six-week radiation protocol terminations, preparations have begun for the journey home. The first of these families goes home tomorrow. We go next Thursday. Another six families have started packing and preparing for school. But as we near the completion of radiation, our outlooks and regimens make us feel very far apart.

It seems that in our group there are two types of families. First there are those facing months, if not years, of additional chemotherapy and surgeries. These families have two weeks to one month off to go home, but then they will return for another dose of severe chemotherapy and weeks in the hospital. And while they have the most difficult path ahead, their prognoses are relatively positive. Then there are those who are here for radiation only or combined radiation and chemotherapy treatments. They're going home for good, with the exception of an occasional checkup visit once a month. In some of these cases, the prognosis is still almost 85 percent survival. I envy both. We too will go home after our six weeks and return for only monthly checkups. And while I certainly love being able to take my daughter back home, I'd spend weeks, months and even years if it meant that the survival prognosis would be better than 10 percent. In a way, we are our own class.

Happiness has replaced despair. The same parents who haunted the halls at 2 A.M. every night, unable to find the sleep that they so desperately needed, now compete to see who will go back home first. Dinner is filled with conversations of school, basketball, work and travel. Gone are the endless Internet cancer searches, the bottomless cups of coffee and the pajama bottoms. Still, I don't feel any different. Today is just today, and tomorrow is too far away. Hope is the eternal promise.

Day 52—JANUARY 19

Therapy of the mind is just as important as therapy of the body. Today we concentrated on the mind, and the hospital is no place to start. So after radiation therapy, we set off for another road trip—this time to the largest indoor complex we could find: the Opryland hotel. You see, I had my fill of the museums, the malls and the hallways, and to tell you the truth, I could use a bit of therapy of the mind as well. If you couldn't tell from the journal, my thoughts haven't exactly been optimistic lately.

Obviously the Opryland hotel isn't a young child's palace. You won't find amusement rides, cartoon characters or water-slides, but it was perfect for Elena. She has never been much of a kid to begin with. If given the choice between a roller coaster and a library, she'd choose the latter. For her (and us), Opryland was heaven. From the moment she entered the room she ran to the balcony, opened the doors and declared, "Dad, come look at the jungle!" Then she had to call Grandma, Mom and Allyson just to tell them about her view. And she didn't stop with that— she also proceeded to tell all who would listen that this was "the fanciest place" she'd ever been to.

For the next two hours, all we did was sit on the balcony, drink our exotic waters from the bathroom faucet and offer toasts to the view (thank you to my family for the "toasting" gene). Then after finding out that Mom took a wrong turn in Louis-ville and would not arrive for another two hours, we decided to take a quick tour for as long as Elena would last. An hour and a half later and after nearly six miles, I cried uncle. It turns out she has had much more practice in her therapy sessions than I had back and forth from the room to the kitchen. The walk ended with a race down the "jungle trails" of the hotel, where Elena left me in the dust. And for the first time, she actually ran and felt confident enough to not just walk fast. Balance was always our last hurdle and it looks like we're starting to clear it. Another reason to celebrate.

It turns out that upon learning about Elena, the crew of the Opryland hotel decided to share in our celebration and join in too. Suffice it to say, she was a princess and we were in awe.

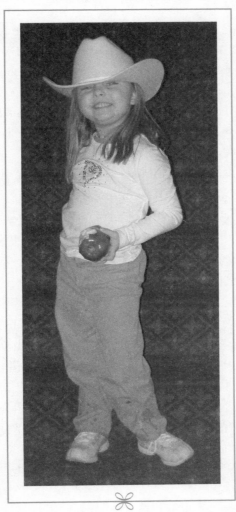

What a way to end a day and what a way to celebrate Elena's return to childhood. Cheers!

Day 53—JANUARY 20

The princesses once again received the royal treatment at the Opryland hotel. It seems the housekeeping staff has adopted Elena, bringing her gifts, breakfast in bed and now custom-fit Opryland robes. This was great, especially considering that both Elena and Gracie no longer fit into their pajamas. There's nothing like having breakfast on the porch with their bellies hanging out and their pants up around their knees. The robes made us look like we belonged here. And at least they had pajamas. In a hurry to get on the road, Brooke forgot hers and spent the night in jeans and a T-shirt. Thankfully, they gave her a robe as well.

For a day we forgot about Elena's condition and tried to be a family. It didn't work, of course. Gracie wanted attention, Elena fought with Gracie, and Brooke and I had forgotten what it was like to have another parent around. Brooke says we need to relearn how to be a family. I know she's right. For the past two months, we've been in different cities, each with a child that we can't discipline or another one we won't. The result was a lunch we spent chasing Gracie and Elena, all while struggling to have a conversation. I know that this will change when we get back together next weekend, but I also know that we desperately need some independent family time with just the four of us to get back to living. I fear that otherwise our lives will become even more chaotic with the passing visits of family and friends. And while the support is welcome, we also need to find our own way. Even though we've spent three days together, Brooke and I have not been able to speak to each other uninterrupted for more than five minutes. It will be nice to see her again next weekend if the situation allows.

Day 54—JANUARY 21

Yesterday when we went to the mall, we visited an outdoor adventure store. We saw kayaks, bikes, snow skis and rollerblades. Normally this would have been a store to dream in, however, under the current circumstances, I did more soul searching than dreaming. It took walking through that store, hand in hand with Elena, for me to realize how much we never did. Elena and I talked about kayaking. Brooke and I have always wanted to kayak with the girls and dreamed of buying two-person kayaks and taking the girls with us on tours of waterways and lakes. Now I realize that summer may never come soon enough. We looked at the bikes and I remembered our bikes gathering dust in the basement along with the trailer we bought last year for the girls. I think we got one weekend out of the bikes before getting wrapped up in "more important" things. I looked at the snow skis and realized that Elena had never been snow skiing, let alone even experienced snow deeper than six inches. I realize that this time is lost. All the things I planned to do with her are now fading and I may never have that second chance.

Will we have the opportunity to do these things? I hope so, but I will never know. And there, in the store, as I turn to Elena and explain to her about snow skiing, she tells me, "Maybe next year, Dad—when I get older." That would be wonderful.

Day 55—JANUARY 22

Odds are fine as long as you're on the winning side. But if you're one of the unlucky ones, they're irrelevant. Facing cancer, I think every parent looks to the odds as a way of determining their actions. After all, odds are everything in buying stock, sports and business. Recently, however, I've come to the conclusion that our odds are immaterial.

Let's say she beats the cancer—why? Was it due to the odds?

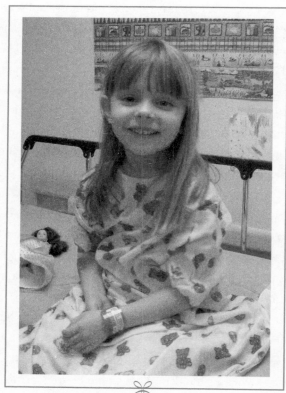

Or was it from our fantastic strategy, her outlook or a miracle? Say she doesn't. Was it because of our horrible strategy, our outlook or Murphy's Law? Maybe it was just a bad diagnosis. Either way, the odds are irrelevant in the final conclusion. And if she's one of the nine in ten who don't beat it, will it even matter in the end? In our mind, that's 100 percent after the fact. Besides that, what do odds mean after you've already lost the odds game and developed cancer in the first place? The way I figure it, we've already been a one-in-a-million shot. But who isn't?

Anyone with cancer makes decisions based more upon their personal attitudes and values than the odds anyway. In Elena's case, we also made decisions based on the moment and on her current condition. Religion played a dominant role as well, although under the current circumstances, we have a hard time turning to religion.

In our short time here, we've met many families: the ones who are newly diagnosed, the ones who have relapsed, but mostly the ones who were beaten by the odds. Every day you're surrounded by the chance to be discouraged and disheartened, but somehow you aren't. And while some may say that the communal lifestyle offers safety in numbers, I know differently. It is facing the impossible that hardens even the weakest soul. We will beat this cancer, we will see Elena graduate, we will beat those odds. I'll take that bet.

Day 56—JANUARY 23

Today was Elena's last radiation treatment. She didn't want to go. But after she was told that she could go home in two days,

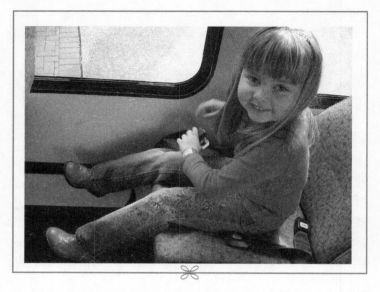

she changed her mind. Unknown to me, this also triggered a long-forgotten memory of a pledge that her mother made to her in Cincinnati, *two months ago*! If she would finish her treatments, Mom would buy her pink cowboy boots. At the time, I'm sure it was a good idea for Mom, but for me now, this would begin a journey of many miles. I'll spare you the details, but the results are a new pair of pink cowboy boots to match her pink cowboy hat. Suffice it to say, it took five stores to find size-ten pink boots. Hey, what else did I have planned for the afternoon? Thanks, Mom. Two can play this game. I told Elena that if she comes back and completes her MRI with Mom in two weeks (they'll be here for just two days, and without a car), Mom will take her out that day and buy her a stuffed purple unicorn with wings. Good luck with that one. It's about as difficult as pink boots.

Day 57—JANUARY 24

There's a tradition at the house. At the conclusion of their stay, every resident gets to leave their handprint on the walls of the kitchen. For the past eight weeks we've cooked under these colorful tributes, wondering when it would be Elena's turn. That time was today. So with paint in hand, Elena and I made her stamp on the kitchen. Of course, you can guess what color she chose—pink and sparkles. And in true Elena fashion, she had to do one better with a photo of her as well. Ultimately, I ended up doing most of the artwork as the staff decided that her space would be on a post eleven feet off of the ground overlooking our kitchen. With Elena's newly found fear of heights, this meant a quick lift in the air to stamp her left hand and then directions from the ground up to Dad on the ladder.

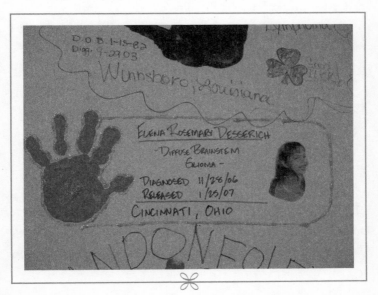

And just like all of the other kids before us, her name, diagnosis and date, and the date of release were imprinted on the walls. Unfortunately, many of the other kids had abbreviated "date of diagnosis" as "D.O.D." and, knowing how I interpreted that for the first week before I figured it out, I was not about to use the same abbreviation. I'm not quite sure how we felt about cooking in a kitchen filled with memories. Some days the handprints were uplifting. And although we could only find three other diffuse brain-stem gliomas in the kitchen, these showed us that we were not alone. Families wrestling with the same fears and hopes had also cooked in this kitchen and even burned most of their food as I had. Then again, it always ended with the thought of how many were left. About that point, you gave up cooking and went to the table without the last course. The green beans just weren't that important. As a result, I always had a ten-minute rule. If I couldn't prepare it in less than ten minutes, I wouldn't do it. Ten minutes was all I cared to reflect on. Of course, I don't know if I even spent ten minutes in my own kitchen at home.

By the time the imprint was finished, it matched Elena perfectly. Pink, sparkly, beaming and simple. Good-bye kitchen—hello home.

Day 58—JANUARY 25

Today we left the house, hopefully for good. Not that it was a bad place (ask me again when I'm cleaning everyone else's dishes for the millionth time in the communal kitchen), but we

didn't like what it represented. I gave Elena the option of stay-
ing another day and leaving early Friday morning, but she felt
as I did, and we ran to the car immediately after her radiation
appointment and started directly home.

Sure, this won't be the last time we'll visit the hospital. There
will be monthly visits for prescriptions, checkups and MRIs from
now until she beats this disease, but each of these trips will be
confined to a day and a plane flight back and forth. And hopefully we will never stay more than three days ever again.

Fifty-eight days down and it seems like a lifetime. I wish it
felt even longer. And through that time you never forget. I always
thought it was just a line when people told me that they never
stopped thinking about life-changing events such as this. Now I
know better. You think about it getting dressed, brushing your
teeth, reading a book, working and especially when you tuck her
in at night. Every minute is not an exaggeration. They also say
this was the easy part—that radiation is the simplest part of the
process. That part is now over and I wonder what is next. From
here, you wait and see.

We've given her a lifetime limit of radiation and now it is
up to the miracle. Radiation has given us time to understand,
respond and react to the disease; that is all. Now we find out if
our reaction is the correct one. In the best of scenarios, radiation has cut the tumor in half or even completely removed it.
But every doctor tells us that even if it is gone, it will come back
with time. That's where the experimental chemotherapy comes
in. Hopefully this is the magic bullet and we will never utter
the word "relapse." With relapse comes desperation and even

more uncertainty, for radiation cannot help then. My new favorite reading is *Clinical Oncology,* a 1,400-page manual on cancer. Knowledge is our crutch.

Today the clock starts and we look to remission as the goal. Now we are on our home turf.

GRACE iLOVe GRACE GO GO!

iLOVeto
MoM

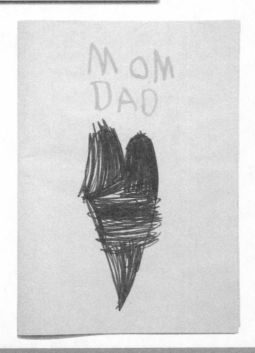

MOM
DAD

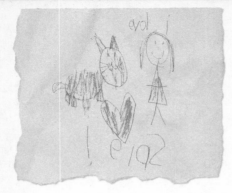

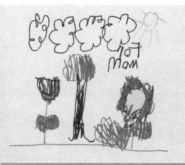

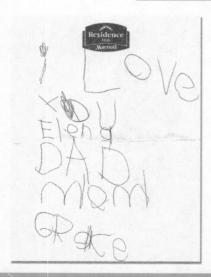

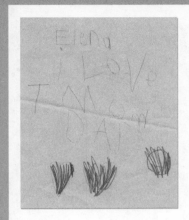

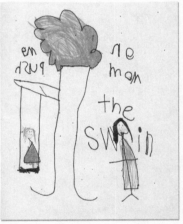

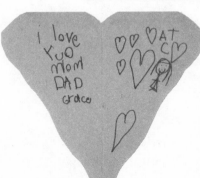

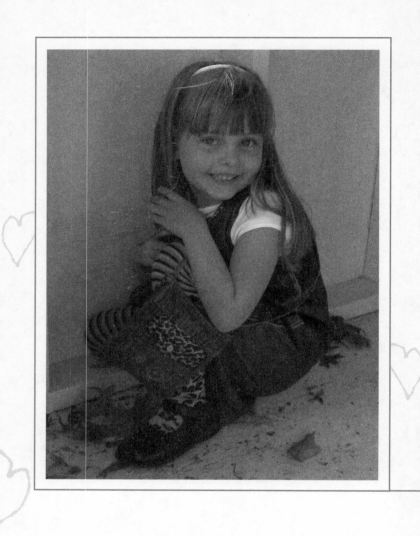

part 2: the honeymoon

Day 59—JANUARY 26

L AST NIGHT EVERYONE slept well. When we awoke, it was normal. I went to work, Elena and Gracie went to school and Brooke went for show-and-tell. Hey, someone had to help haul the seventy-nine photos, radiation mask and sticker chart.

After dropping Gracie off at preschool, they headed to kindergarten for the big presentation. There they were greeted by a four-by-eight-foot welcome sign and about three hundred elementary students and teachers. It was everything that Elena needed but never expected. We thought Mom would be the one who cried, but we were wrong. It was Elena. Thankfully kindergarten was calling.

By 2:30 P.M., it was time to pick her up. Well, maybe not quite, but I was tired of working. I quickly resumed my role as an overprotective dad and roamed the halls outside her room. Finally, after one hour of waiting, she was ready. I think I beat the rest of the students out the door as I tucked her under my arm and ran for the car.

This evening, we went looking for stars at the local observatory. There she saw the moon, stars and probably would have even seen Saturn if we had been able to stay up past 9 P.M. That's all right. My star is home tonight asleep in her own bed. Mom and I will sleep well tonight.

Day 60—JANUARY 27

How do you go about living your life knowing what you know? More and more I wonder if modern medicine is a godsend or a curse. While we appreciate the advances and cures it delivers, at what point do you fear the anxiety it creates? I know this anxiety firsthand, the uncertainty and fear. So what is a normal life? On any other Saturday we would have started it with a lazy wake-up at 7 A.M., had breakfast with the girls and then proceeded into a litany of errands, house cleaning and home repairs. Sunday was reserved for family. Time was plentiful before—or at least so we thought—and our priorities were different. Cleaning, errands and repairs were more important than time with our children. These were our guilty pleasures and now there is no time left to waste.

You see, every action, every decision, is now weighed against severe consequences. Need to take a shower? Make it quick— you can save five minutes there. Need a haircut? You can go for another month—wait until she's asleep. Need to clean the house? That's what the night is for. Life is about them and nothing else matters.

When will it end? Will it ever end? Who knows, but I hope I have to keep making these decisions for the rest of my life. That's the curse of medicine. You can diagnose the disease, but God keeps the time frame secret. I guess it's best this way to keep living and to see importance in every action. I see it now but only hope that the lesson will soon be over and she will be cured. Until then, every weekend, afternoon and morning will be different.

Day 62—JANUARY 29

Cereal kiss! That's what I get every morning before I leave for work. It's Elena and Gracie's way of sending me off and I can still feel the Lucky Charms residue on my cheek. First I get a normal kiss and a hug as they lull me into a false sense of security. Then, just as I'm about to leave, they run from the table and ask for one more kiss and hug. That's when I get the milk-laden kiss and they run back to the table chanting, "Cereal kiss! Cereal kiss!" before I can catch them. They think I'm fooled, but the truth is I can't wait. Okay, maybe the first couple of times, they tricked me, but it didn't take long to catch on.

It's these moments that a parent enjoys most about having kids—not even the trips to Disney World (although this is also fun), the first day of school or even birth are quite as exciting as the little daily moments. From age four through eight is the sweet spot. This is the time that I feel is the most rewarding as a parent, when you watch their creativity and personalities grow.

Of course, I also thought two through three and zero through two were the sweet spots. Maybe it just keeps getting better.

I keep reminding myself of this as I savor every day with a new perspective. Reminders such as "Wash your hands—use soap" and "Wash your hands—use water" no longer frustrate me quite as much. A little, but not as much as before. Who thinks that as a parent they have to tell their children, "Stop pinching the banana," "Don't lick the butter" and "Don't brush your sister's butt with the toothbrush"? As if using a hairbrush would be any better. And to think I used all of these phrases today alone. I guess that's what being a dad is all about.

Being a dad is about more than the good and the bad, it's also about taking the time to treasure what you have and finding the humor in everyday life. Without it, you'll never make memories. It's true; I don't think I'll soon forget the image of Gracie licking the butter out of the jar.

Day 64—JANUARY 31

How do you measure time? When Elena asks how long she'll have to go to the doctors or have her blood taken, I reply "a while." Is "a while" a couple of months or will it be for the rest of her life? And what if a couple of months are the rest of her life? "A while" doesn't mean the same thing it did yesterday and I hope that one day "a while" will mean a lifetime.

As I walk through a day, I hear comments such as "I wish my children were older," "I wish it was summer" or "I wish this day would end." These offhand comments are how we relate to each other and how we grapple with time. But to me, I want it to just be today. As a matter of fact, I'd like it to be yesterday. Time has a way of sneaking up on you even when you don't want it to. I only wish it would also slow down.

A trip to the grocery store isn't the same. I not only shop for price (or organically grown), but I've also started to shop based on expiration dates. These dates have new meaning when you think that the food you're buying may last longer than your daughter. There's another reason to like organic foods: no preservatives, so they expire in a week.

For now, the clock keeps going as we struggle to respond. I know the answers will come soon, but for now, we wait and fight the urge to react. This is Elena's time. Her days comprise school, tickle time and lots of bedtime reading. (Tonight, the bedtime reading lasted an hour. It's certainly helping her reading skills. Brooke and I can no longer mouth out the letters to "needle," "blood" or "hospital" without her knowing. I guess fear helps the learning curve too.)

How long until the cure? I don't know, but I hope it's less than "a while."

Day 66—FEBRUARY 2

Today was the day of bridal dress shopping and Elena's aunt was more than willing to oblige. It's actually her wedding, but considering the circumstance, it was all Elena's day. For six years we drove past the local wedding dress store on the way to day care, and every time, Elena would proudly announce which one she would wear when she got married. So it was only fitting that when Keith asked her what she always wanted to do after being released from the hospital, she responded with "I want to buy a wedding dress." From the beginning we knew that this was going to be a tough day for Keith and me, but it was what Elena wanted. Luckily, with her aunt's wedding, we also had the occasion.

Thankfully we found a wonderful wedding dress shop that was nice and quiet—the perfect place for two kids strung out on sugar.

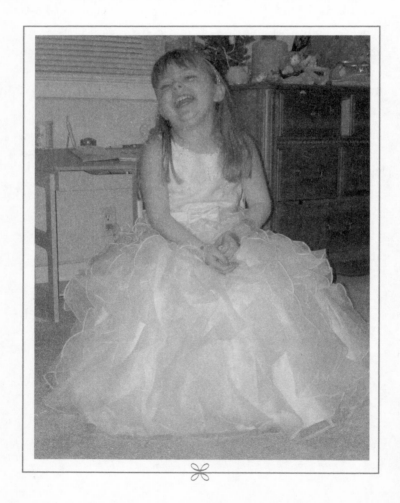

We started off by having the girls choose the dresses they wanted to try on. And the only ones left were either too large or lime green. After finding the best of the best, we knew it was impossible to have the flower girls wear the same dress. These girls are so very different and not one dress fits all personalities. Elena chose this pink, sparkly, ostentatious number that said, "I have arrived!" Gracie, for her part, chose a white number with pink flowers and tulle draped all around that says, "I am demure and dainty and belong on top of a wedding cake."

They twirled and pranced around, helping their aunt try on her own dress. Gracie helped by entertaining the boys in between the dresses. Bounding in and out of the curtain, she would announce the color and type of each dress, promptly falling back to the floor as her feet got caught in the lace and satin. We couldn't stop laughing at this little girl in a beautiful, fancy dress falling all over herself, every time saying, "I'm OK!" Elena was in charge of announcing the entrance of her aunt and giving us an update of the time remaining until the next dress appearance. She was our coordinator. Grandpa, on the other hand, was in charge of Keith. Luckily, he was there to teach Keith how to behave while a woman tries on clothes. Saying, "That dress looks like a pinwheel," "You could wear that to a disco party" and "That's my third-favorite dress" are not the ways to a woman's heart—especially one who is about to be married in the dress of her dreams.

While Keith was unable to muster enough tact or patience for wedding dress shopping, every dress his girls tried on was "perfect," "beautiful" or "That is the princess dress." And when it was all over, I noticed that price was no object where his girls were concerned.

Day 68—FEBRUARY 4

What do you do between the big moments in life? Is life made up of TV shows, small talk and business? Or is it instead made up of charity, accomplishment and leadership in service? Do we ask our children, "What do you want to be when you grow up?" or should we ask them, "What do you want to accomplish when you grow up?" And what is the total value of all the time we spend on diversions and distractions rather than the true purpose of living? Can one person change the world? Can one person cure cancer?

Too often the answer was no, but with Elena I've come to see the world differently. When this began, we were nothing but spectators, content to watch the world affect us. Cancer isn't new to our family—quite the opposite—but you never understood it, let alone participated in the cure. Instead, you prayed for miracles and waited. And while prayer has its place, too often we ignored the reality that miracles also occur in people as well. After all, cancer was the doctor's job. What did we know about cures, foundations and tumors? We were accidental victims and life now affects us in ways we could never have imagined. After having spent the past sixty-eight days in bewilderment, we start to see our responsibility in the destruction of this deadly disease. And just like Elena isn't, we too are not powerless, insignificant or immune to this challenge.

Last night I spent the evening paging through clinical trials and working through another two hundred or so pages of my clinical oncology manual. Some things I understand, others I do not. Some parts seem logical, but others seem flawed. I am an uneducated mind in a sea of unknowns. I do not profess to understand or even be able to help remedy what so many much more highly educated people continue to puzzle over. In a way, I guess awareness is part of the solution. The more we are aware of characteristics of this disease, the more we will begin to understand our roles. I trust that time will be on our side.

Day 71—FEBRUARY 7

It was time to go back to Memphis for a checkup. This is the next stage of the disease. Every MRI from here on out brings the hope of remission. Today was not one of those days. Not to say it was negative, but it wasn't positive either. It was what was "expected." The tumor was reduced about 50 percent by the combination of radiation and chemotherapy. And while this is a positive direction, it is tempered by the reality that radiation is over and chemotherapy is our only option to keep the tumor at bay. Now it is a battle to keep the tumor static and avoid a relapse. This is the new standard.

In analyzing the tumor, the doctor also notes the presence of "specks of blood." And while this, by itself, does not mean much, with the potential for bleeding, our recommended protocol list is reduced from sixteen to two. I guess more research is in order.

Elena and I decided to do our own preliminary research tonight as we loaded the MRI CD copy into my computer so we could view the "head disc," as Elena called it. This was an unexpected release as we ended up lying on the bed in fits of laughter. Elena was laughing because she could see her entire eyeball in the scans. I was laughing because it was ridiculous that I even began to think I could find the "bump" in those scans, though Elena kept prodding me to show her the bump.

After playing doctor, Elena decided that since we were ordering in pizza for the night, she was going to serve me. She laid out hand towels for the place mats, pulled up the chairs and gave me a menu. She served me the pizza and asked me to wipe my mouth because "this is a polite restaurant." Apparently, she isn't a busboy though, because I ended up with dish duty. Thank goodness it was all paper and plastic.

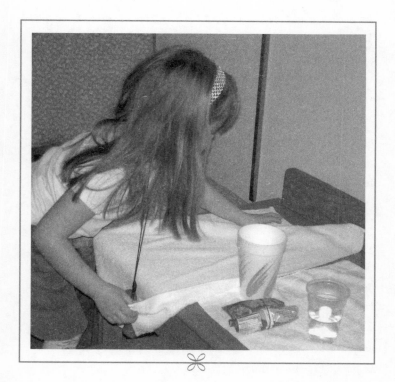

Day 74—FEBRUARY 10

Today was our pre-Disney day and the girls couldn't be more excited. Six months ago we planned it in conjunction with a business trip. Now it's everything but business, and we'll be accompanied by both sets of grandparents, my sister's family and Brooke's brother's family. In our own way, we're a convention all by ourselves. So Brooke and I were preoccupied with the task of cleaning the house and packing for every weather event and every emergency that could arrive. After six bags, we finally gave up and figured we'd buy the rest if we still needed it.

Day 77—FEBRUARY 13

The grandmas were playing for keeps today. That's the problem with combined family get-togethers. Inevitably, the result is a "Fight-to-the-Finish Grandmother Contest" where the gifts fly as hard as punches. From the left comes gummy candy, from the right come books. Soon, the competition turns ugly, with stuffed animals, firework-inspired desserts and jewelry. And before we know it, the girls are spoiled beyond our best corrective efforts and there's no way to fit it all in a suitcase. Today was no different. Luckily, Brooke and I brought a fourth suitcase with this in mind. Hopefully it won't get any worse. Though I know it will with Valentine's Day around the corner. Already I can see the love message hearts and the dolls arriving on the doorstep. And just when we're trying so hard to go organic and get antioxidants in her.

Today was a soaker in Disney World. So we spent the day

in It's a Small World (I know you're singing the song now—good luck getting it out of your mind) and the Haunted Mansion. Thunder Mountain would have to wait for another day when it was dry. By 4 P.M., the crew was ready for drier conditions as we headed to the luau at the Polynesian Resort. There we were greeted by leis and much-needed alcohol and food—in that order.

For the first time, we sat together as a group of fifteen and talked, laughed and ate. It was a lovely ending to the day and a wonderful way for Elena to enjoy her loving family. Then as the sun dropped and the temperature cooled, Elena asked to sit on my lap to watch the fire dancer show. Of course I could not resist as I watched her eyes twinkle in the light of the performance. To be honest, I have no idea what happened during the luau; I spent the next hour admiring and holding her.

It was the longest she had sat with me since she was just months old without squirming or running to Mom and I was

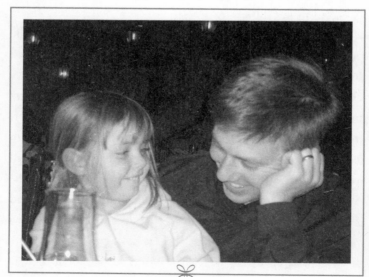

not about to give her up. When it ended and it was time to go, I picked her up, laid her head upon my shoulder and continued to the ferry that would take us home—never mind that my arms had fallen asleep thirty minutes ago. And when we returned, my arms ached, but so did my heart. For despair forces you to live in the present while your mind races to the future. Regardless, tonight I was the luckiest father around.

Day 78—FEBRUARY 14

Elena's never been what you would call "outgoing." She's never volunteered for anything, let alone a challenge. She won't sing aloud in the car or the bathroom, she won't talk to strangers and she won't try new food. For her entire six years, her comfort margin has been restricted to what she knows and what we force her to do. Then, and only then, will she admit that it was a good idea in the first place.

After the experiences over the past four months, we never expected anything different from her. She'd still resist and we'd continue to prod. And we were right. What we didn't expect, however, was how extreme it would become. Since her diagnosis, everything has become a challenge as she fights to remain in her comfort zone. And unlike before, this is now accompanied by tears, screams and a fear that we have never seen before. After four months of needles, surgeries and paralysis, her confidence was tattered and the only way to fix it was by force.

For nearly an hour today, Brooke and I attempted to convince, bribe and cajole Elena into going down a waterslide with her cousins. But we had no such luck, so after thirty minutes of pressure, I pulled her close and began the climb. After ten steps, she pleaded for me to stop; ten more steps and she cried that she had to go to the bathroom; ten more steps and she complained that her right foot hurt; after the final ten steps, she told me that she was afraid of heights. I was not going to get the Father of the Year award this year this way.

Finally, I did what any caring father would have done in my position—I pushed her down the slide and watched her turn the first corner screaming. Then I jumped in behind her and followed. I think they call that "forced fun." And although I knew that she did not want to go, I knew that she needed to try.

No sooner had she reached the pool than she was on her way to the top again, telling everyone she met along the way how brave she was to try the waterslide. No confidence problem this time—she beat me to the top and even the fear of heights seemed to be cured. Forced-fun parenthood is severely underappreciated. Tomorrow we will work on the other rides. Enough for today.

Day 82—FEBRUARY 18

Today we board a plane for home. Yesterday the grandparents, aunts and uncles left, giving us one day to be a family of four. Still, that brings us no comfort as we're left with our thoughts. This entire vacation has been a struggle against time. Every ride brings a hope that it will never end. Every parade brings the chance that the floats will continue to appear. Every fireworks display comes with the wish that the lights will continue to float against the dark sky. But just as the rides, the parades and the fireworks come to an end, so must this vacation. For us, these endings are more than the return to life—they are also one more step in a direction that we do not wish to travel. And as the days click by, our lives become more complicated and our hugs for Elena become more uncertain.

I don't want this vacation to end because of the weather or the experiences, but because I don't want to lose this "honeymoon," as the doctors refer to it. This is the time when she can be a six-year-old again without the hassles of blood tests, MRIs and complex discussions with doctors where we avoid the "unmentionable words" in her presence. In truth, I don't think we could

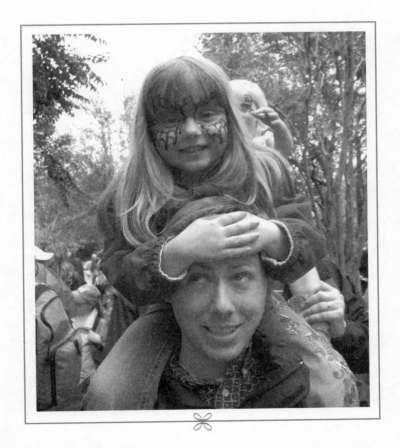

have done any more over these past seven days and I doubt my knees and back could handle much more walking, but my mind could have traveled much further had time allowed. This is the reality of time; it never waits and it never repeats.

Today Elena looked at me and asked if she could get married one day in Disney World. This caused me to stop, look up and wonder to myself. My response was "Of course." I hope this is not a lie and the best answer I could ever give. Let time be on our side for a change and let me pay for that wedding. You are all invited.

Day 83—FEBRUARY 19

Sunflowers are Elena's new passion. Van Gogh's *Sunflowers* to be exact. *Dogs Playing Pool* apparently just didn't have the same appeal as van Gogh. And when we traveled to France this past Saturday (okay, France, Epcot), Elena immediately knew what she liked. There she saw van Gogh in all of his glory—on postcards, on shoulder bags, on cutting boards, on switch plates and on prints. She especially loved the *Starry Night* switch plate, but she decided to settle on the *Sunflowers* print—especially when I wouldn't shell out the $18 for the switch plate. Elena then took the opportunity to share with the cashier that her "grandpa-grandpa (as Elena knows my grandfather) had the real picture at his house" and that this was just a copy. I think we got the cashier's attention at that point, regardless of the language gap. Never mind that the picture that hangs on my grandfather's wall is also a copy of the real thing painted by my great-aunt; to Elena, this is the original.

Tomorrow the print goes to school for show-and-tell, and from what I hear she needs not just one item but two things to share, for this is the responsibility of a "Star of the Week." Brooke and I don't know if this is exactly true, but to be honest, I don't think either of us minds, and neither will her kindergarten class. She can share the joy and beauty of van Gogh with the class as she tells them how her grandpa-grandpa owns the real thing. Yes, there really is a multimillion-dollar painting located in Cincinnati. We, on the other hand, will be plenty satisfied with the $32-million smile it brings to Elena's face. Thank you, van Gogh.

Day 84—FEBRUARY 20

A year ago I had never heard of the Caldecott Medal. Today, I at least know that it is an award for literature. Beyond that I still don't know what it signifies. But to Elena, any book that has won the Caldecott Medal must be special. These are the books we read first before bed. These books even have their own special bookshelf, just so they don't mingle with the "common" books.

Elena loves her books and it shows. In her room you will find three shelves of books, and there are another two shelves in Gracie's room, where wall space is more plentiful. Gracie, on the other hand, loves stuffed animals. She stores these lovingly all over the floor. Elena would never dream of doing this with her books. Each book is placed on the shelf, binding out, letters facing the same way, with a filing system that rivals anything Dewey ever imagined.

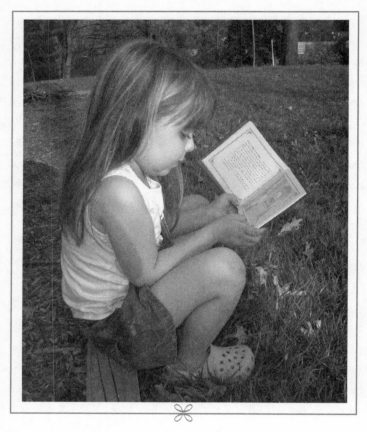

To read a book with Elena is a methodical journey. First, you must do away with the book jacket if it has one. After all, in order to experience the majesty that is bedtime reading you must not only view the pages but feel the cover as well. But be careful to place the jacket back on the shelf— you will need to re-cover it as soon as you finish the book. Next, always remember to mention the author's name, present the cover to the audience and then prompt them to tell you what they think the book is about. Never mind that the audience may only be Mom, Gracie and me. Third, open the book to the first page and review the copyright and the illustrator if different than the author. Now, we must pause at the copyright and discuss Elena's age at the point of original publication. Finally, you are ready to read, but make sure to discuss the quality of the illustrations and how the author conveys movement with the pictures. Faraway pictures that become close-ups indicate that the subject is traveling. It is also important to understand the illustrator's use of color. Bright colors convey happy feelings, while dark colors convey sadness. Once you have made your way through the book, close it, set it on your lap and ask the audience to "discuss the book" with you. Then and only then have you truly enjoyed your bedtime reading. Now you know why it also takes us an hour or more to read three children's books every night.

Every day we learn from Elena. To tell you the truth, I've never looked at a copyright before or examined the colors of illustrations. While I am the parent, she is still the teacher. So when 7 P.M. comes around, it is time for us to sit in a circle Indian-style and listen. This we do well. When you ask her what she wants to be when she grows up, she tells you she wants to be a mom and then a teacher. And with her prodding, even Gracie now wants to be a teacher instead of a "police girl." I know that Elena will be an excellent mom and teacher. Until then, I'm ready to be her student for an hour or two every night.

Day 86—FEBRUARY 22

It seems that lately all of our serious conversations occur in the car. Yesterday was no different. At 2 P.M., I picked her up from school for a weekly checkup appointment at the hospital. Immediately, she knew what this meant—a blood test—and she did not like it one bit. This time distractions fell short; she knew my game and wasn't about to be fooled. I talked about her day; she talked about needles. I talked about having popcorn after dinner and a movie; she talked about blue gloves. I talked about kittens; she pleaded to go home instead. And although I'd have loved to take her home, I knew that without blood test results we'd never be able to stay at home. Finally, I gave in and tried to reason with her. I explained that blood tests allowed her to go to school, come home to Cincinnati and be with her friends, and that these blood tests were part of the reason that she was getting better.

"But I am better, Dad," she responded. Yes, she was better, but just as it took a long time for the tumor to grow, it would also take a long time for it to shrink. This she did not understand. After all, she could walk, talk and eat, so why did she have to keep going to the doctor and taking the medicine? "Am I ever going to get better?" she asked. "Will the bump grow back and make me use the wheelchair again? I'm eating good food and taking the medicine, so it goes away." I paused. She waited. She asked again. "No, every day it will get better, but it will take a lot of time and a lot of trips to the doctor." I promised myself I was telling the truth. These trips, these tests, the medicine and her patience would ultimately win out over this disease. The rest of the trip was silent. No distractions could change her mind this time.

Tomorrow I hope our conversation is more about kittens than our uncertain future. Regardless, it's during these times with Elena that I learn the most. She is both smart and painfully aware of her circumstances. I often wonder if she's avoiding the discussion as much as I am. Maybe she thinks I just haven't figured it out yet. She's much smarter than we can ever know.

Day 87—FEBRUARY 23

Every step and every word with Elena now takes on new meaning. On Monday it was a slurred word. Tuesday brought a complaint from her about not being able to hear. On Wednesday, Brooke and I decided it was worth a visit to Children's Hospital to see if it was anything serious or if we were just overreacting. We were overreacting. But with her symptoms being as subtle as they were in the beginning and quickly progressing to a full-blown paralysis in a number of days, we felt it best to discuss it with a doctor. I love being wrong. Hopefully we can overreact for the next eighty years.

With tonight came another attempt to overreact as we walked around the mall with Mom. Elena was complaining of being tired and the first thing we noticed was her right foot starting to turn to the outside. Then she caught her foot on the escalator and fell to her knees. For Gracie this would have been normal. For Elena, this was another reason for concern. I carried her the rest of the way. By the time we reached home, the foot had returned to normal and she climbed the steps to get ready for bed. Could I be wrong again?

The doctor says that glioma symptoms frequently reappear in the reverse order of how they improved after radiation. That would mean that the first to go would be the gag reflex, then the right leg and right hand, then the ability to speak and eat. Tonight she sits on the couch with a bag of popcorn—gag reflex fully intact.

Somehow I don't think this will ever change. She will continue to surprise us and we will continue to analyze her every move. I love being wrong, especially now. Seventy-nine and a half years to go . . .

Day 91—FEBRUARY 27

Next time the swim instructor will know better. And maybe, just maybe, when she tells Gracie to jump out into the pool into her arms, she'll take a step back first. Second thought—maybe she'll take three steps back.

Today our pursuit of physical therapy brought us back to the local pool. We enrolled Gracie and Elena in swim classes. And while we'll never be able to go every week with Elena's continuing treatment schedule, we were anxious to inspire Elena in the midst of the wintertime monotony. Gracie was just an added benefit— call it "competitive drive" for Elena. And there, on the edge of the pool, their lesson began. To assess their abilities, the first lesson was jumping into the pool. In response, Elena eased her way to the edge, ever so careful to avoid slipping, tripping or actually getting wet in the process. First came the toe, then the leg in pure hokey-pokey style. The teacher moved forward. "Jump into my hands," she said. Elena sat with her legs dangling and stretched out her arms. And in what seemed like an hour, she finally leaned forward and ever-so-gracefully drifted into the pool.

Gracie was up next. For this, the teacher figured that if the older one took this long, then surely the younger one would need more prodding. She took a step closer. Gracie waited with

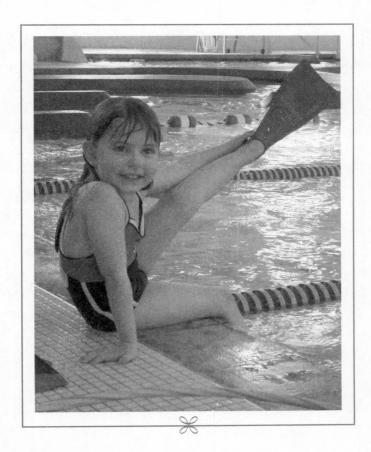

her back against the wall, fooling the teacher with her patented bashful look. For anyone who doesn't know better, this comes across as shy and timid. To everyone else, this is the look of scheming and mischievous intentions. The teacher did not know Gracie. "Come on, jump into my hands," she implored. Gracie didn't need prompting and she sure wasn't going to ease into the pool. After all, in Gracie's world (we call it Graceland), this was permission. And with that, she bent forward in a sprinter's pose, pushed off the wall and took off for the pool—too late for the teacher, who tried to step back; but Gracie was already in midair. And when she landed, Gracie made it not only to her hands, but also to her chest, her head and the hair the teacher had tried so hard to keep dry. Oh, and the form! Legs and arms up, belly down. It was the perfect belly flop, so perfect you would have expected her to continue skipping across the water until she reached the other side. She didn't of course, as the teacher was blocking her way. Instead, they both went under with Gracie on top. Suffice it to say, I think she passed this portion of the lesson, no matter that she still can't swim.

You don't realize how much Elena has lost until you see her swimming. Before her diagnosis, she'd swim across the pool unaided. Now she can barely manage twenty feet with a kickboard. Funny how one month of paralysis can do so much damage. But I guess that's why we are here. The more she practices, the more she builds muscle to help her through the rest of this battle.

Day 92—FEBRUARY 28

A dad's job is to protect. This is what I would tell Elena, from her first trip down the playground slide to her first MRI. It was my motto, and if you ask Elena what a dad's job is, she could tell you without hesitation. No matter what happened, Dad would be here to save and protect you. And I believed it. It is a simple job. I defeated bullies, darkness and nightmares. I believed that my hands were quicker than lightning and my skin tougher than armor when it came to protecting my daughters. No matter what the threat, I told them that their dad would be there to keep them safe. Little did I know what lay ahead.

And somehow through the beginnings of this disease, I thought that by possessing the powers that come with fatherhood, I would somehow be able to protect her once again. I would be able to cure cancer or find the miracle doctor who had the solution but just didn't know how to tell the rest of the world. That power today is now quickly fading as I come to grips with our declining options.

Today we learned that her chemotherapy protocols may not be as positive as we might have hoped. We're not totally sure, but with a trip to Memphis in the cards for next week, this will be our single biggest issue. The implications of such a result are discouraging to say the least. The drug that we have pinned all of our hopes on may have zero to little impact on the growth of the tumor in combination with radiation; this is according to another patient on the same trial who met with his doctor last week. Simply put, we might have wasted the best opportunity to beat this tumor. Now all we can do is pray for chemotherapy, but with her radiation lifetime maximum dosage already exhausted, this is a long shot at best.

And so today a new fight begins. A fight that we must understand and prepare for, and ultimately win. And while the time and direction that we must travel will ultimately be decided by the disease alone, as a father I take little reassurance in knowing that we are doing all we can do. Elena's time for miracles is upon us as the medical community is losing options daily. But just as a dad's job is to protect, it is also to never give up. And while inside I want to stop, I can't. The cancer may grow, the side effects worsen, but I must still protect. Cancer has scarred my family before; this time must be the last. Still I feel that somehow I should have seen it coming. I should have done more. Protection is more than just about the fight; it's also about prevention. And in this way I have already failed. Never again.

I plan on keeping the promise I made over six years ago when I held her for the first time. A dad's job is to protect.

Day 93—MARCH 1

Gracie and Elena are more than just sisters, they're also best friends. With only twenty-two months between them, they share more than clothes, toys and hobbies; they also share their lives. This was the way Brooke and I intended it from the beginning. Having both come from families where we were three or more years apart from our siblings, we felt that our children would benefit from being two years apart or less. Little did we know how right we were.

At twenty-two months, Elena had no idea how much her

life was about to be impacted, but she did know she was now a big sister. Proudly wearing her "I'm a New Big Sister" pin at the hospital, she took to her duty as bottle feeder as she gave up her room and her toys for the new addition to the family. And although they would play with each other and spend hours on rug patrol in the family room, we soon realized how much they would come to love each other the day we heard Gracie laugh for the first time. Around six months after her birth, we found Gracie giggling in her swing while Elena danced and made funny faces in front of her. It's never been the same since. Now Gracie returns the favor daily with her staged antics and infectious smile.

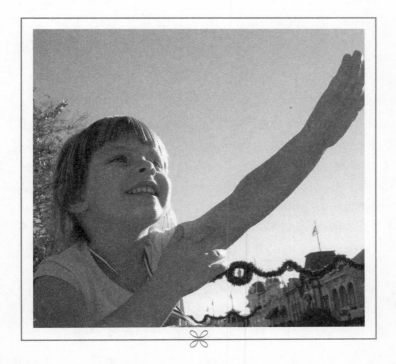

Even today, Gracie is the comedian while Elena is the comforting mom. Just this morning while Gracie was upstairs in the midst of a temper tantrum over her clothing selection, and Brooke and I had all but given up, Elena quietly climbed the stairs to calm her sister. Five minutes later, she came downstairs holding Gracie's hand remarking to both of us how wonderful Gracie looked this morning, while Gracie wiped away tears. Not only had she managed to calm Gracie, but she also dressed her in the exact clothes that we had failed to get her to wear twenty minutes earlier.

Friends don't have to be the same in order to get along. Sometimes it is the differences that make a friendship work. In Gracie and Elena's case, it is also what makes them perfect for each other.

Day 94—MARCH 2

We call them "rusty eyes." It's the moment in the morning that you wish you had gone to bed earlier the previous night. For most people this lasts until the first cup of coffee or after the morning shower. For Brooke and me, it lasts all day and into the next. And it's more than just a lack of sleep; it's a weariness and exhaustion that have become our lives.

After the diagnosis we couldn't sleep. Night after night we'd try, but from midnight to 4 A.M., we'd look up at the ceiling wondering how to wake up from the nightmare. Now it's different. Now we can sleep but don't want to. This is the new norm. Whenever we aren't working, eating or spending time with the girls, we're reading e-mails from other parents, researching on the Internet for protocols or reading our stack of oncology materials. And by the time 11 P.M. comes around, we've only gotten started. So we continue in our desperate search for options. The doctors tell us to enjoy the honeymoon. Other parents of previous DIPG children tell us to prepare. We want both. There's always the looming question of "why her?" That's where faith comes in. But instead of questioning through faith, we choose to have faith that the solution will present itself, and so sleeping is not an option. The "rusty eyes" continue, night and day. This is our God.

Day 95—MARCH 3

Sometimes things just happen. Without reason—without consequence. Sometimes every day doesn't have a moral and isn't neat and tidy. Yesterday was one of those days. It started with our family on opposite ends of the country. Gracie was still sick at home after recovering from a cold. I was making my way home from California from a business meeting. Mom was home with the girls, struggling to balance business and family. Elena was at school suddenly feeling tired and overcome with headaches. Everything else could wait for now.

By noon, Brooke had received a call from kindergarten that Elena was tired and missed Dad. But upon picking her up from school, she also discovered that Elena was suffering from severe headaches. And after three hours of trying to force liquids, treating with Tylenol and allowing her to sleep, the headaches only got worse. It was then that she decided to make her way to the emergency room.

One hour later, Elena's condition worsened. Her right leg started to drag again, her voice became garbled and her right hand was less than perfect when put to the test. It was not good news. And by the time I arrived, three hours late thanks to airport delays, an MRI was already in the plans. The good news was that she went through the MRI on her own, no sedation, no problems. The bad news was that the tumor had grown in the last month. We are now in what they call a "recurrence"—the end of the honeymoon.

To understand what this means, you need to understand what we expected. From the beginning, we were told to expect recurrence anywhere from three to seven months from the end of radiation. In time, this was upgraded from seven to fourteen months from diagnosis, as we met with more-specialized doctors. Even at the worst, we expected the tumor to possibly come back in late April. At that point, we would have had enough time to evaluate alternatives, assess results and spend time with our daughter—if you can somehow believe that three months from radiation is enough time. And if it grew, somehow, it would be small growth. We received nothing of this sort. One month from the conclusion of radiation was not nearly enough. Worse yet, the tumor didn't seem to be growing by small amounts or even affected by the chemotherapy. Nothing can convey our feelings and I won't even try.

Where do we go from here? The most promising protocols need weeks to formulate and I doubt we have even two weeks to work with. The fact is we didn't work fast enough. Our options are limited and our understanding of this disease is minimal. We may have just missed our best chance to beat this cancer.

There is so much more work to do, both for us and for Elena. We need more time. The chance for miracles is today and the cure starts now. Tomorrow may be too late. I love you, Elena.

Day 96—MARCH 4

Welcome to the "gray area." The experts cannot tell whether the growth in the area is swelling from radiation or actual progression. Our team determined the increase was small enough to call it stable. Elena also woke up with a fever and a headache on Monday, so perhaps all the symptoms were caused by getting sick, rather than the swelling. We'd love to believe that that was all. Next month we have a follow-up MRI, so we will be watching that very carefully. We also got a go-ahead on our nutritional plan for Elena. As long as it is natural, we can give it to her.

Today during lunch, I think Elena discovered the diagnosis for her headache. "Mom, I had three weeks without a headache and one week with a headache." Brilliant. For three weeks, she was taking her chemotherapy meds. This week she had an "off week" where she didn't take meds. Perhaps these are the withdrawal symptoms!! I have an e-mail out to our doctor to find out if I need to enroll her in medical school. Every day Elena amazes me with her intelligence and ability to simplify the most complicated situations. And while she's still working on her MD, she practices doing the nurses' job every chance she gets.

Today, while receiving her monthly port flush through an IV tube, she calmly informed the nurse that she had missed a bubble in the syringe and she should elevate it and squirt a little bit of liquid out of the top to clear it. The nurse looked at me, looked at Elena and then looked at the syringe. Elena was right and there was no doubting it. As if to assist further, Elena gestured at the syringe the nurse was holding just in case she did not clearly understand her. "Wow, she certainly is perceptive, isn't she," the nurse commented as she cleared the syringe and continued. I asked her if she wants to be a doctor or nurse when she grows up. I don't think I have seen her shake her head "no" faster. Maybe we can still convince her to cure cancer before moving on to becoming a soccer player.

Day 98—MARCH 6

Abnormal. That's what they call Elena's tumor. Normally the thought of having an abnormal tumor would strike fear in the hearts of parents. After all, "abnormal" conjures up images of instability, deviant growth and untreatable conditions. And while some of these may even be correct, for us, "abnormal" also means hope. You see, "normal" brain stem gliomas have a poor survival rate—no treatment protocol and plenty of despair. So being "abnormal" must certainly be the opposite of despair—right?

From the beginning, they've referred to her tumor as abnormal, and while "abnormal" breeds uncertainty and fear, it also gives us hope that somehow this is a tumor that no one has ever seen before. Yes, we are actually hoping that this is a tumor that *no one has ever seen before*. Imagine that.

Maybe, just maybe, "abnormal" will also mean that it is curable. Surely the 10 percent of children who survive this disease must have also had abnormal tumors. One can only hope.

Day 101—MARCH 9

For the last couple of days, Elena has been talking to truckers. The voices haven't been clear, but occasionally we make out a song or an inquiry about traffic coming from her Hello Kitty walkie-talkie. A CB radio might not be the best toy for a six-year-old, but we always figured that she was picking up signals from a kid down the street. That is, until she took the walkie-talkie with her on our trip to the home and garden show. A mile down the interstate we finally connected the dots when the signal became clearer and her questions of "Who is this?" were met with names like "Tina Ray," "Big Mac" and "Diesel Duo."

Little did they know that the person on the other end was using a $25 Hello Kitty radio and couldn't care less about the southbound accident at the bridge. Nevertheless, Elena kept on talking, asking questions and relaying traffic information as we passed the truckers heading northbound. Like a rancher herding cattle, she directed them to the right and then the left lanes, no matter that she had no clue as to which lane was closed up ahead. Traffic probably took an extra hour that night, thanks to our little girl. And by the time they discovered it, I planned on being out of range.

Day 102—MARCH 10

I'll never look at a hot dog the same way again. Only after you are fighting for your child's life with just a pot and a spatula as weapons do you start to really fear the contents of everything you put in your mouth. Every night I spend at least an hour or two reading about nutritional strategies for Elena. Anything natural is fair game and the list of beneficial foods is endless.

It has now become a fine art of trying to stuff as many "goodies" into a meal as I can. Rice and veggies are cooked in green tea to sneak a bit more into her diet. I have become skilled in cutting shiitake mushrooms into millimeter slices to hide them in her dinner. The whole mushroom-hiding thing is especially hard because Gracie is horribly allergic to mushrooms. I wind up cooking two separate dishes so Gracie doesn't break out into hives. Elena caught on one day when I lunged to snatch a plate from Gracie when she sat at Elena's chair at dinner.

Some nights I long for my convenience food, my Rice-A-Roni, my chicken nuggets, my fifteen-minute meals, my school lunches, my dinners out without scrutinizing the menu and my sleep! I hate having to ask the grandparents to take back the candy they brought for the girls or ask my brother not to order the hamburger for his daughter because Elena would want one. But then I realize that if this is the only battle I am fighting right now, I will take it. Next week is rosemary tofu with leeks sautéed in garlic and lemon zest—yum!

Day 103—MARCH 11

Today was the beginning of Elena's wish trip, and this time she wants to go back to Florida. Two weeks after her diagnosis, the wish coordinator called offering Elena the opportunity to do anything she wanted to do. But facing an uncertain future, neither she nor I wanted to talk about wishes. She was offered

the world—swim with whales, go to the real Eiffel Tower, anything. But after another two weeks of discussion, all she could
settle on was to swim with dolphins—and that was with Gracie's
input. I guess it just goes to show you the simplicity of Elena's
wishes. And although I realize the value of this simplicity at a

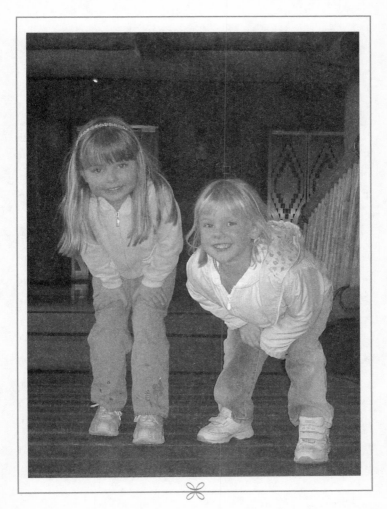

time in her life when control is critical, I can't help but wonder if her concept of vacation will ever expand beyond Florida. With the Grand Canyon to the west, whales to the east and plenty of ground to cover, would she appreciate these more if we took her elsewhere? After all, she has been to both Disney World and SeaWorld before. Still, this is her trip and for now it is an easy trip given the circumstances. She has never been swimming with dolphins before so at least this will be a new experience. Tomorrow will be the best day ever for sure.

For Brooke and me, the vacation takes on a different meaning. This trip brings on feelings of hesitation and melancholy that are accompanied by pure and total exhaustion. I realize this now as I am too tired to sleep and too hungry to eat. But instead of craving cookies and my pillow, I yearn for the moment when Elena's in total remission and I can rest. The moment I can stop experiencing every second of life and live it instead.

Our trip to Orlando is particularly significant as this is our last planned vacation in our foreseeable future. Precancer this was not anything special; we never took enough vacations and never planned for them more than three months in advance. But now, with the possibility of this being Elena's last vacation, I'm so apprehensive that I don't want it to begin. After all, if it doesn't begin, it can never end—right? Two weeks ago, Brooke and I came to this realization as we stood on the deck of the train station at Disney World for the last time before leaving the park for home. There we realized that it's impossible to stop time regardless of how much you love your children. You take pictures, dry the tears, relive the moments and hope that you never forget. But at the end of the day, you look forward, stop thinking and keep moving, for that is the only way to survive. This is ultimately what it's about when you deal with a terminal illness; you deal in the present and you never stop for fear that you will never get back up. And then tomorrow, you begin all over again. It's a type of exhaustion that you can't rest from and a feeling you will never forget.

This time I want the vacation to be perfect. So far, it is. Not one frown, not one tear, not one missed moment. This is the impossible mission, but the mission nevertheless. Life is about living and I know this. Living is about both the good and the bad. Living is about the present. We will live when we are at home and we will live when we are in Orlando. For us, it is every minute until we ultimately fall asleep at the computer or at the foot of her bed. We can do both in Orlando just as well as here. Bring on the dolphins!

Day 104—MARCH 12

Dolphins feel like giant rubber bands. At least that's what Elena says after swimming with them. Although she insisted that yesterday was the best day of her life as we sat waiting for Daddy and Gracie, she let me know that today was the best day of her life and that this is what she had been dreaming of. I have to admit, this was in my top five days as well. There is nothing like holding my daughter as she experienced one of the most amazing adventures of both of our lives.

The day started with standing in line to get our passes and

Elena endlessly asking, "Can we go yet?" I think that voice was stronger today. Then when waiting for the photographer to take our picture; "Can we go yet?" Then they took us on a tour of the park; "Can we go yet?" We got fitted for wet suits and masks; "Can we go yet?" When we finally reached the edge of the coral reef, with snorkel gear in hand, and took the first step in the water, Elena screamed, "I don't want to go!" The water was a frigid 72 degrees—too cold even for pasty white Ohioans on spring break. So after about five minutes of Elena wailing that she was going to freeze to death, she got used to the cold and found a new topic to whine about—"I don't want the fish to touch me." I figured now wasn't the time to remind her that she was three hours away from having to touch a four-hundred-pound fish. After ten minutes of convincing, we snorkeled in the depths of the two-foot sandy area to see two-inch guppies. Fifteen minutes later, we were floating and

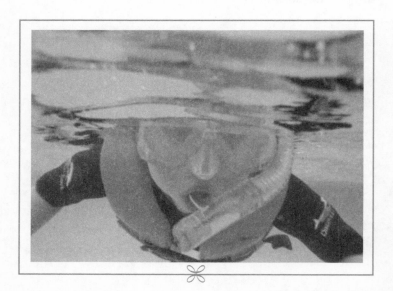

skinning our knees on the "seafloor" as we made our way out to the deep end.

I am sure we were a sight with two little girls flailing, screaming and riding on the backs of Keith and me as we desperately tried to swim in fifteen-foot depths with no life jackets. But then, something magical happened, as Elena suddenly became a snorkel queen. Even though when she saw the stingrays, I could hear muffled screams through the snorkel, she kept her head down and headed in the opposite direction. On the other hand, when I saw the stingrays, I ripped my mask off and wildly swam to the shallow end. Elena was back in her element. In Tennessee, Elena would swim for hours without tiring, and today, she was as good as new.

After a bit of lunch and Gracie grooving to the sounds of the lunch buffet reggae band, we were off to the dolphins. Unfortunately, Gracie wasn't old enough to swim, so this one was for Elena and me. As we inched into the water (because it was still a chilly 72 degrees—again, not as warm as you think!), the dolphins starting swimming and splashing around. Elena then said, "Look how excited they are; they must know I like dolphins so they must be excited to see me!" The trainers told us tidbits of information on dolphins while Elena ignored them and squealed in delight as she got to pet the dolphins, Coral and Roxy.

Next was the dolphin ride, and this was one activity of which Elena had no fear. Coral decided to take Elena on the long trip and instead of going straight to the trainer, she zigzagged through the water to make the trip last longer and Elena loved it! Only after we were done did I realize Keith and Gracie had disappeared. Apparently, Gracie had to go to the bathroom right before the

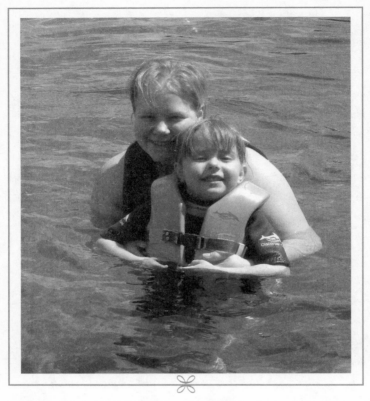

dolphin experience started. Obviously Dad was a tad disappointed. Luckily they had a professional videographer who captured the moment for only $50 plus tax.

That night over a dinner of ice cream, we recounted the experience of a lifetime and then returned to the hotel to enjoy our video of the swim. Then I tucked Elena in and she whispered to me, "This is everything I wished for." Enough for me.

i love
you Mom
Elena

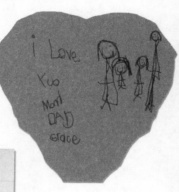
i Love
you
Mom
DAD
grace

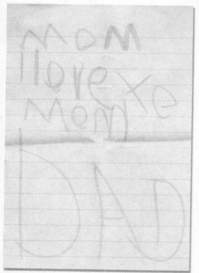
Mom
I love you
Mom
DAD

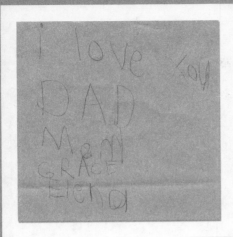

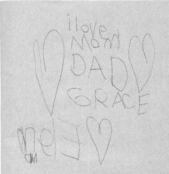

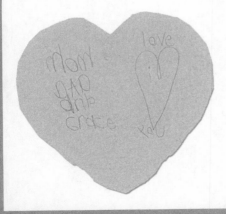

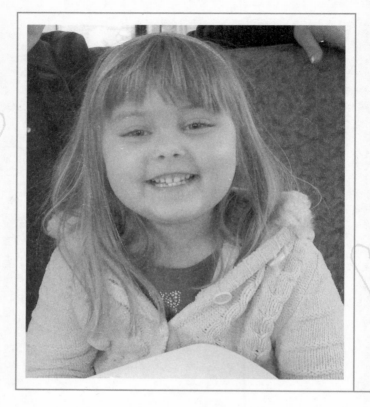

part 3: life after progression

Day 107—MARCH 15

THEY SAY THAT Elena's symptoms will not vary. The doctors say that when she experiences a muted voice and difficulty walking it will be constant and unwavering. Today I had to wonder. After a spectacular day yesterday touring Disney, Elena awoke this morning with a whisper and trouble with her feet. At first we thought she was looking for attention so we ignored her hand signals for more juice and forced her to talk. She tried, but we could tell she was having problems. Coincidentally, today is the third day after her last dose of steroids.

Brooke says I'm wrong to expect that Elena will fully recover. That a muted voice and a slight limp should be the least of our worries in the face of this type of cancer. The worst part is that I know she is right. Still, there's nothing harder than seeing your child be the victim of something you and she cannot control. As a father, nothing short of perfect health is acceptable in your child.

After all, isn't that the gift of childhood, perfect health and a lifetime of opportunity? And now Elena is being robbed of both.

Still we stay positive and focus on the present. But Elena knows better. Every morning she rises with a smile only to succumb to depression when she climbs out of bed and remembers that her foot doesn't work the same as before. This is more evident than ever as we share a room with her on vacation and see her respond to these difficulties. And when she turns to us to say good morning, her smile quickly turns to sadness when she has to instead pantomime her morning greeting because we can't understand her words. From there the day brings depression and frustration as she tries to eat breakfast, tries to tell us what she wants to wear and what she wants to do. And by lunch, she's tired, aggravated and angry. By dinner, she can barely eat and only wants to go to bed. Not because she can't eat but because she just doesn't want to fight it anymore. Tonight was one of those nights as we struggled to keep her up past 7 P.M. and keep her stomach full. She ate one egg and half a sausage today. Every other attempt was met with tears.

This is certainly not our most difficult battle and both Brooke and I know that we are only at the beginning. But how do you tell a six-year-old to keep going when all she wants to do is stop? We let her make daily choices such as her clothing, her activities and her food in an attempt to give her back some control, but even this is met with tears. Tonight we could care less about organic food and just wanted her to gain back some control by eating anything. Fast food would have been enough. She refused and instead chose breakfast at Denny's. But even there, we had to force her to eat more than three bites of her egg.

Today was not a good day; hopefully tomorrow will be better. And with the rain coming into town, it looks as though our trip to kayak with the manatees may be canceled. Today the beach was good, but with high winds and 70-degree temperatures, we barely spent thirty minutes on the beach in the sand before retreating for the warmth of the hotel room. Not what we had planned, and considering her frustration, it is not what she needs right now. Comfort, relaxation and control are the keys to her regaining her self-esteem.

Day 108—MARCH 16

Elena has always been the nurturer and Gracie has always been the entertainer. When it came to babies, puppies and kitties, Elena's brow would scrunch up in awe. As for Gracie, she never took notice; she was never interested in anyone younger than she was or anything of the furry persuasion. After the diagnosis, Keith and I had serious concerns about how Gracie would take the inevitable increase in attention toward Elena. Gracie has always craved the spotlight and Elena was happy sitting on her own doing drawings or reading her books. But fate had forced both of them into a realm they were not accustomed to and did not enjoy.

After three months of the new environment, Elena has learned that she simply has to smile and hide behind Mom or Dad, and eventually the attention will shift elsewhere. With Gracie, she was still struggling with the new norm.

As Elena's weakness began to grow in her right side today, Gracie has become the best of both personalities. After a full day of Elena being pushed around in the wheelchair, being given the front seat on the roller coaster and being given a taste of cotton candy, Gracie walked through the entire park, asking Elena if she liked riding in the front and even thanking Elena for sharing the cotton candy.

When we returned to the room and Keith and I began to pack while the girls got ready for dinner, we overheard a very eye-opening conversation between the "ladies." Elena was fretting about getting her hair combed and going to dinner. Gracie very calmly spoke to Elena in the quiet controlled voice of a skilled negotiator. "Don't worry, Lena. Mom can put your hair in the ponytail so it doesn't tangle. Do you want that?" And she continued, "Do you want to pick the restaurant tonight, Lena? I will let you pick out the restaurant so that you can eat what you want. Will that make you happy, Lena?" She even offered to hold Elena's new coveted Shamu lunch pail while Elena struggled to get into the van for dinner.

Gone is the bickering—okay, the constant bickering—and now we have two very grown-up little ladies. We always looked at Gracie and pondered whether she would ever grow up with her silly antics and infectious laughter, but she has done it much faster than we could have imagined. She has taken over the role as big sister in light of Elena's condition. I am in awe of the selflessness she has displayed on this trip. She knew this trip was for Elena and not once did she complain that we weren't doing what she wanted. Only tonight did Gracie nicely ask if we could do pirate putt-putt at home, when our planned trip to the enticing miniature golf in downtown Orlando was called off by Elena's exhaustion. Tomorrow we go back home.

In some ways, I am grateful for the new enlightenment and

the hope that Gracie will be able to handle the increased focus on
Elena. In other ways, I fear how this new, grown-up Gracie may
handle whatever is to come. In some ways it was easier to have the
girls bickering than to have them so dependent on each other. In a
new world where our girls are forced to grow up beyond their ages,
I'm proud to have them as my own.

Day 110—MARCH 18

Four months ago, "tickle time" was our only nighttime ritual. This was the time at the end of the day when I connected with the girls and chased them up the stairs to bed to tickle and tuck them in. Gracie would always play the victim, acting like she tripped on the stairs just so she would be caught first and get the most tickles. Elena, never shying from competition, would race to be first in bed and then heckle Gracie over her victory. Then at the end of the night after closing the doors and turning off the light, she'd call out for me and calmly inform me that Gracie had gotten more tickles than she had and she was due since she was the first one in bed. Of course, I always obliged.

Tonight our nighttime ritual involves much more than just a simple tickle and a kiss. First we must read. Junie B. books are still the favorite, as long as Mom is doing the reading. My responsibility instead is to now offer foot massages. I guess I don't need an accent for this duty. Of course, we can't forget Gracie, so I get to do two more feet. I'm waiting for the day that Brooke asks for hers as well.

Then there's the holy water. For the first month it came

by the gallon. And while I never professed to be the most religious person around, I can't help but believe that this also has an effect. And with four types of holy water from places I didn't even know existed prior to this entire religious experience, we have quite a selection to choose from. So we move from bottle to bottle, sometimes using all four types, depending on her mood during the day and our emotional state. How to apply it I have no idea, but I figure it's best to get it close to the tumor, so on the back of her neck it goes. Tonight, for the first time, Gracie noticed and now she also gets a dose of holy water on the back of the neck. I wonder how long it will take before she wants Elena's chemotherapy treatments as well.

Last but not least, there's tickle time. And as always, Elena is the first in bed. Gracie still falls on the floor just so she gets caught first. I often wonder if this is the most effective treatment of all. I know that it is the one I will never forget. You see, a successful treatment should be about more than just treating the tumor; it should also be about treating the patient. And nothing brings a bigger smile to Elena than a dose of tickle time. Of course, it also brings a smile to me as we connect once more. Sorry, Gracie, Elena was first.

Day 111—MARCH 19

The sign language has returned. With Elena's voice becoming increasingly congested and her vocal ability decreasing, she is back to resorting to hand signals and spelling. And while she has been able to hide her right-leg weakness pretty well, it's her speaking and gag reflex that we're worried about now. Meals are no longer simple since portions must be cut into small bits and she has started to avoid hard foods for fear of choking. And while we're not quite at ice cream and applesauce, it is discouraging to say the least. Both Brooke and I pray this is still swelling and not progression. With the MRI scheduled for the first week of April, we will soon know.

Day 113—MARCH 21

Our life has become a web of contradictions. A paradox of what is and what we know to be. It was a beautiful day. Sunny, warm and just the hint of spring stirring from the bulbs unearthed by our home's remodeling project. Any other day it would have been perfect. Brooke and I took advantage of the opportunity and left work early to pick up the girls. From there, we went home to enjoy the waning afternoon hours pushing the girls on the backyard swing and playing "Old McDonald's" fast-food drive-through in the windows of their playhouse. This marked the first time we ventured into our backyard since late October, when our lives were much simpler. And right now we needed a taste of that. Elena and Gracie climbed, swung and practiced penny drops, while Brooke and I longed for ignorance, bliss and idealism. They, along with their friend, ate graham crackers and released their pet butterflies into the air, while I watched every step that Elena took with concern and fear. We hoped the limp would just go away and we'd be left worrying about mosquito bites again. No such luck.

Today Elena's mood improved, but her condition deteriorated. The limp and loss of voice worsened and it was now joined by a slight headache, drooling, trouble swallowing and double vision, all symptoms we've seen before. And while we're still working under the assumption that this is the result of swelling, we increasingly have to come to grips with the reality that it may be progression and our time frame may no longer be a matter of months, but weeks.

People ask us how we're doing. We tell them, "Fine," but today that will no longer suffice. They ask again and we know then that they want the real answer. Then we shake our heads, shrug and utter, "You know." Still the truth is that they probably don't know and we don't want to be reminded. So we go on with our days and find solace in routines. It's the simple things that keep us going. Folding the wash, emptying the dishwasher, holding meetings, calling customers; these are distractions we can hardly concentrate on, but distractions that allow us to function. And for a minute or even an hour your mind stops focusing on the future while your heart never stops reminding you of Elena. How are we doing? Fine, as long as we keep going. Fine, as long as Elena keeps going.

Tomorrow, "fine" will not do. Elena is scheduled for another MRI. This one was not planned. With her recent symptoms, our hunch is that the tumor is growing. Where do we go from here? If it is a progression, do we stick with the chemotherapy? And if we don't, what options do we have? Other protocols may not be available for another month, so do we go a holistic route? Starting today, no options are favored because no one knows. This is the part of medicine where it stops being about science and starts to verge on faith. Still, what is faith? Is it faith that we will make the right decision or faith that it is in God's hands? And while we can't just walk away from the decision, we are increasingly realizing how little impact we have on Elena's situation and how much we just can't solve. I'm not satisfied with this, but it just doesn't matter. Once again, we have little control and this is what I must accept. Yet in some way I know that Elena could accomplish so much more if given the opportunity, and I pray for this chance.

Ultimately, we will make this decision and it will probably come tomorrow. Beyond that, God will show us the way. Hopefully He will also give both Elena and our family the opportunity to do more for this type of cancer in a way that cures it for all children. All we ask for is time and guidance. Sunny days don't come often enough.

Day 115—MARCH 23

So this is how it feels. I got a taste of it when they first broke the news to us of Elena's tumor about three months ago. Of course we didn't believe a word of it. When they told us last night that the tumor had nearly doubled in size, we went through denial, anxiety and anger all over again. Only this time it was real. This time, I looked around the room but couldn't see; I heard what they were saying but never understood; and my writing was blurred as my hand shook with fear. And during the entire consultation, all I could do was tell myself to look serious, concentrate and breathe. Somehow I would begin to understand. Somehow it would all make sense. Yes, the tumor area had enlarged, but what it meant I had no idea. Sadly, even today, after spending the entire evening last night reading everything I could get my hands on, I still feel no more confident in our decisions.

Now we need to also examine Elena's quality of life. Do we risk it all and go for yet another cure, regardless of her condition? Do we go the safe route and try the drug that gets another week but we know will not work? Or do we give up on medicine, provide comfort and try the natural route? Sadly, we never predicted that we would need to make this decision now. Not with our daughter and not before the start of the window they gave us when she was originally diagnosed. But this is an abnormal tumor and this has meant a perfect storm of cancer. The worst tumor, the least understood, growing in the worst place at the fastest speed, exceeding all expectations. I'll take normal any day right now.

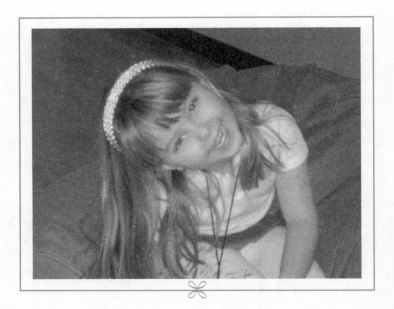

Where do we go from here? On Monday, Brooke and I will be faced with a decision that we can't fathom and are not prepared to make. The experts tell us that they just don't know, while everyone else tells us to follow our hearts. I've been listening, but my heart isn't talking. All it does is ache. I had always thought "heartache" was an expression. Now I feel it every day. It is an emptiness in your chest that you try to fill with work, shallow humor and sometimes food, but the reality is that you'll just learn to ignore it over time. Right now, I keep trying to fill it with hope, but every time I do, doctors who tell us that they too cannot find survivors immediately dash our hope. Whatever happened to the 2 percent survival rate? Was that merely a psychological lie designed to allow us to sleep for the past three months? If so, why not make it 98 percent instead?

So now we make a decision based on no numbers and no information. If we believe it is swelling, then we should stick with the chemotherapy. If we're right, she'll have a few more months of survival. If we're wrong, she'll be lucky to last two weeks. If we believe it is progression, then we switch to a new drug regimen. If we are right, then she may last another month. If we are wrong and it was truly swelling, we'll lose the few months we would have gotten if we stayed with the previous chemotherapy and get a couple of weeks instead. And while each option is a matter of weeks, they are precious weeks. New treatments and possible cures come out every day and it is only a matter of time until *the* cure is tried on a patient like Elena. So in the long run, even one week can mean a lifetime.

The decision is ours alone, but for now we take advantage of every moment.

Day 116—MARCH 24

Today I spoke with another father. His son died one year ago. And now he is a member of an exclusive club—a club for parents who lost their children. So now he fights for a cause where before he spent time with his son at baseball games, doing homework or teaching him to ride a bike. In doing so, the cause has filled his life and a void. It will never replace his son, but to him it's about saving the next child.

He tells me that the second-worst day of his life will be when everyone forgets about his son. Today I can't even begin to think about this. I'm not ready for this and I don't want to join this club. I don't want a cause, I want my daughter. Somehow I doubt that I will have either the resolve or dedication to fight this fight if I ever lose my Elena. For me it is about her and nothing else. And while I hate the tumor and despise the cancer, it will never be as personal as it was with my daughter. Maybe I'm wrong and maybe one day it will be me on the other end of the phone, but for now I listen and learn.

So we talk about research or the lack of any. It seems that just like for us, for parents before us the cancer too was personal and more about their children than a cause. And when they lost, the disease gained. The surviving family moved on, researchers found other specialties to study and a child was forgotten. And now, today, with Elena we are left with few options. So I now talk with another dad about the second-worst day of his life rather than the hope of saving just another life.

It's not anyone's fault. It truly isn't. We can't do this alone; it will only work if we work together. But I'm as guilty as anyone else. And I still don't know if I can stand to help. Right now all I can think about is Elena. And in this regard I am powerless.

Instead of talking about forgetting our children, let's start tomorrow talking about remembering them and their sacrifices. They are not victims—they are fighters. Elena is and so are hundreds of other children fighting this battle daily.

Day 117—MARCH 25

It is all about the quiet moments now. With Elena's voice still quite weak, whenever we are around a large group of people or around strangers, Elena withdraws into her shell. She will nod her head and that is about it. She knows she can't speak above all of the voices and that strangers can't figure out what she is saying, so she says nothing at all. In one of those quiet moments she asked me why I don't let her paint the walls. I am not sure where it came from, but I could certainly change that. So with four pure white walls in our playhouse crying out for decoration, we searched for old clothes.

I never realized what a girlie girl we have until Elena stood crying in her bedroom because she didn't want to wear old clothes. She wanted to look pretty. After convincing her that it was only temporary, we set out through the puddles of mud in our backyard and made it to the playhouse Dad made back in the days when we had free time. We opened cans of bright colors and the girls set to work. It only took about ten minutes before the girls tired of painting, so Mom hurriedly painted flowers and birds and clouds to finish the empty sections. The girls put their handprints all over the walls and then we ran back inside to clean Elena's hands of the pink paint that was giving her fits. And to think we would have given her every wall to paint if she only had the time.

Day 118—MARCH 26

The emotional roller coaster continues. And while Elena's condition is improving every day (thanks to a healthy daily dose of steroids that would make even a baseball player blush), we are continually reminded of the uncertain future. Starting tomorrow, we expect the paralysis to return and the voice to weaken as we start to reduce the dosage to a manageable level. Once achieved, we fully expect that this dosage will continue for days, weeks and hopefully months and years to come. Moodiness, bloating and sleepless nights will worsen as the effects of steroids take hold.

With the MRI indicating tumor swelling/growth, we received a call from her doctor with his impression of the film. This much-anticipated call was a source of worry not only for Brooke and me over the decision ahead, but also for every grandparent and relative who called us hourly for a status report. And somehow we figured that this call from Elena's doctor would put our minds at ease.

What we didn't anticipate was a call telling us that they felt that the interior of the tumor *may* be growing, but that it may also be dying. Essentially, the dead portion of the cell mass expanding could influence the growth that we may be seeing. Don't ask me how this is possible, that's what we still have yet to decide, but needless to say, it significantly changed the equation. So now we have an opinion that it might be progression and another opinion that it may be radiation causing dead cell growth or necrosis. Now we're squarely in the middle. A tough decision just got tougher. Tonight will be a long night.

Day 119—MARCH 27

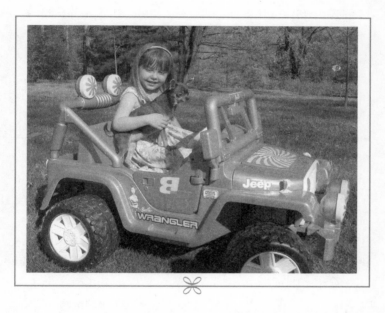

How much does one smile cost? Exactly $229 plus tax. And you pick one up from the toy store in the bike isle. But make sure to bring a big truck to haul it in because you'll need to fold down all the seats to fit this smile in the back of the car. Then prepare for "some assembly required." Smiles take lots of bolts, nuts and miscellaneous pieces to put together. Of course you'll have the customary extra screw and bolt, but don't worry, you'll find out where they go soon enough when you take the smile out for a test drive. Three hours later, there it will be. And for the rest of the day you'll bask in its glow.

I caved. It's purple and pink, has four wheels and has a battery to help it move. It's a Barbie Jeep and it's exactly what Elena always wanted. Even with the steroids, I managed to induce a smile or two. Too bad I lost the camera after recording them. Hopefully I'll find it tomorrow, otherwise that smile will get more expensive.

Too many times this journal has been used to record the "last" things instead of the "first" times. I guess when you go through a struggle like we are, as parents, you start to think in this way. You start telling yourself, "This is the last time she'll visit her grandparents' house," or "This is the last time she'll go to Disney World," or "This is the last time she'll go to *The Nutcracker*." In a way, this is how you prepare yourself for the worst. Then, if the worst happens you won't get hurt. If it doesn't, you'll be surprised. Either way, the pain won't kill you.

Still, it's this daily mind-set that ruins hope and lives. Instead of talking about lasts, we have to start talking about firsts. After all, the first three years of her life were all about firsts: her first step, her first bike ride, her first words. Why can't this time also be about firsts: her first dolphin swim, her first fancy dress, her first waterslide? It's a much better way to think about life, if you can do it. It only requires hope.

Tonight that hope was challenged by reality. It's day three since the news and Brooke and I still haven't made a decision on our course of action for Elena's therapy. Not because we can't or because we don't have all the information. Actually we have more than enough information and plenty of expertise coming from all sides. We find ourselves in the unenviable position of deciding Elena's fate. Worse yet, not one opinion has an edge on the other one. So where do we go from here? No change might be the best course of action.

In light of Elena's recent recovery resulting from her steroid regimen (she now walks, talks and swallows much better), we might decide to take a "wait and see" attitude and reevaluate next week. That's when we'll make our monthly trip to Memphis and have the benefit of a fifth MRI. Perhaps then the decision will be clear and another week of steroid dosage reduction will give us hope of swelling. There's that hope thing again . . .

Day 120—MARCH 28

Dad's a fool. Smiles are free. While he needs a Barbie Jeep, I get them for free all day, especially today. You see, reading this journal you'd think Elena and Gracie are Daddy's girls; not so. In this household it's still very much three versus one. Daddy still gets the punches and I get the kisses. Take today for example: Gracie cuddled and scratched my back, while Elena practiced her therapy with right-handed punches to Dad's stomach. One day he'll learn that kisses work much better than tickling. Until then, Elena gets her daily therapy session. I can see this coming in handy with her eventual boxing career.

Today Elena was genuinely happy. And except for when Dad had to drop her off at school, everything else went well. Lately, Elena has developed a strong attachment to both Keith and me in the mornings. The result is an emotional good-bye at the schoolhouse door. It's not that she doesn't want to go to school; she loves school and can't quit talking about it when we pick her up. It's that she doesn't want to let us go.

Tonight as I prepared her for bed, she told me that she didn't feel that we spend enough time together as a family. I agreed. But I also know that Elena loves her friends and her teacher too. Trust me, dropping her off is one of the toughest parts of the day for me as well (although I think I handle it much better than her father, "Mr. Mush"), but I know that this is just what Elena needs to come out of her shell. In a way, it has become more than just an education but also a bit of emotional therapy. For us, it is a chance to return back to life as well, as we pretend that all is normal and just like it was four months ago.

Day 122—MARCH 30

We call her "Steroid Sally." She's up and down all night, perpetually shy, incurably hungry, and irritable. Last night Steroid Sally started out the day early. More specifically at 12:10 A.M. It was my turn to sleep in Elena's room.

I went to bed at 11:45 P.M. She was up at 12:10 A.M. ChapStick was the emergency of the moment. Suddenly she remembered that she had left her ChapStick in her pants from the previous day and she needed to get it out *now*! For my part, I had just reached the deep sleep stage. My logic was fuzzy, my memory was worthless. And before I truly awoke, I had already walked halfway down the hallway in search of her jeans from last night. Ten minutes later, I found them and returned to her room to find her sound asleep in bed. So much for this being an emergency.

At 1:30 A.M., she was back up again. This time she sat up

calling my name from across the room. "Dad, Dad, *Dad*, *Dad*, *Daad*, *Daddddddd*!" I was awake. She said, "I need my plain skirt." I heard, "I feed my trained bird." Obviously this wasn't why she woke up again. And she doesn't even have a trained bird. She said it again, getting increasingly frustrated with her limited voice and my poor attempts at reading lips in the dark. After the fifth or sixth time, I finally got it. Still, a plain skirt didn't seem like enough of a reason to awake in the middle of the night. I reassured her that we would pick a plain skirt in the morning. Two minutes later she was back asleep. I was awake for the next hour.

At 4:18 A.M., she was up again. This time she sat up, called my name and said, "I have to tell you something." I sat and listened. She said nothing. I walked across the room, wondering if this time it was about a plain shirt or a penny in her coat pocket. She said nothing and instead turned to rest back down on her pillow. The next sound I heard was her snoring. Great, now she was not only waking me up, but also having a dream about waking me up. Just like her mother. Who knew it could be genetic? I gave up and switched off the alarm. Someday I'll actually use it.

Mom's up tomorrow night. But by then, the steroid dose will hopefully be reduced and she'll again start to sleep through the night. Either way, we'll take it. Good-bye Steroid Sally.

Day 125—APRIL 2

Hope comes in many forms. Today it came in the form of a limousine. This time it was a white one. And to think we were expecting a school bus. At school on Friday, Elena's teacher asked if we were ready for Monday. Little did I know that the entire school staff had plans for Elena's first day of spring break. When the limo arrived at 10 A.M., we didn't know what to expect. And after a six-point turnaround in our thirty-foot-wide street with a forty-foot limo, we were on our way.

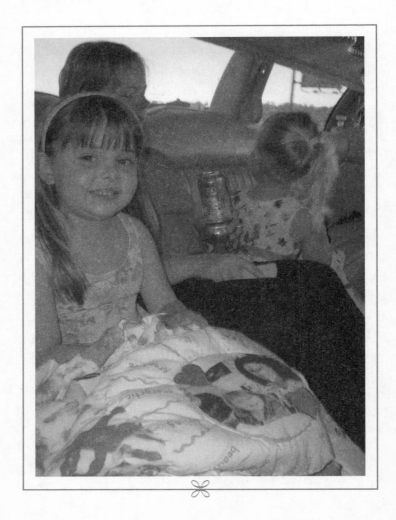

Along the way, we not only discovered clues to our afternoon, but I also discovered my family. We found Elena's hidden laugh, Mom's tears and Gracie's love for gizmos in a limo. If there was a button to push, she pushed it. If there was a drink to drink, she drank it. And every seat not occupied called her name, at least for ten seconds. Thank goodness Mom found the seat belts.

Soon we had arrived at our first destination: the art museum. Immediately, Elena recognized it as she turned and told me that she had been there three times before. This was the fourth, and since the museum is normally closed on Mondays, this time she would be the only guest allowed. Knowing that Elena would be at the hospital for the remainder of the week, her teachers pulled some strings to get the museum to allow a solitary visit on Monday. And so, dodging the army of custodians, floor refinishing crews and curators, Elena received a personalized tour of some of the museum's most prized possessions. There she saw American art, contemporary art, sculptures, impressionist art and even multimedia art installations. She also spent a little quality time with her friends Vincent and Pablo, as she now calls them.

Back in the limo, we learned that a picnic at the park overlooking the river was up next. But not any picnic meal would do; in our case the teaching staff had prepared an organic lunch for Elena, in a traditional picnic basket, no less. Apparently, they had studied Elena's packed lunch selections over the past month and meticulously purchased all of her favorites for this special picnic.

Our memory of the day was beautiful weather, fine art, a perfect picnic and time with our family. And as we prepare for our trip to the hospital tomorrow in anticipation of news that

Brooke and I do not want to hear, we find ourselves bolstered by the support of Elena's teachers and classmates. You see, what we also found in the limousine was a handcrafted quilt made by Elena's teachers and classmates. A quilt of love and support designed by a community that we are proud to call our own and emblazoned with the handprints of every student from her school. In a way, this was the true art of the day and enough by itself.

It was hope, a hope we desperately need and a hope that we must continue throughout Elena's life every day until she is a hundred years old. Regardless of our setbacks and regression, we realize that today we had more than a family of four in that limousine, for covering that quilt was a community of hundreds.

Day 128—APRIL 5

I've never had a hero before now. Sure, I've had role models and even mentors, but I can't say that I've ever really had a hero. In my mind, a hero was always someone who epitomized strength, courage, integrity and an ability to do the impossible. And now as a father, I have a hero in my own daughter. Her strength and courage throughout her treatments have been nothing short of amazing. Throughout the past four months, she's seen her speech, walking and feeding abilities disappear, only to have them return and now disappear again. Still, her resolve has never faltered and her courage to continue smiling seems endless. Her integrity is without question—Elena has never been able to lie—and her concern for others in the face of her struggle is miraculous. All I can hope now is that she will do the impossible. She will overcome yet another hopeless regression and she will triumph over the disease that has taken so many others. Then she can help others to triumph in this struggle with the impossible.

That's the dream and what my hero is capable of achieving.

Day 135—APRIL 12

One hundred and thirty-five days ago, our lives changed forever. One hundred and thirty-five days ago, I sat in the dark holding her hand in the ICU ward. One hundred and thirty-five days ago, they told us that she had three months and six weeks to live. One hundred and thirty-five days. That was when we started a journal for Gracie that would tell the story of her sister. Today is one hundred and thirty-five days from that day.

One hundred and thirty-five days tells the story of a girl and her family, a family involved in a struggle that we fear, but one we hope never ends. Tomorrow we will start a new journey and most certainly a new phase. On November 28 we began stage 1: distress. This was when we first learned of the cancer and discovered medicine's inability to cure her. Stage 2 brought anger: anger over why it was our daughter and how this was allowed to happen. Stage 3 was when we learned to fight. And with countless books on oncology and early-morning Internet searches, we truly began to understand this disease. Stage 4 brought desperation, fueled by the information we had collected.

It's something to feel overwhelmed by the complexity of the disease, but it is another thing to feel powerless in the realization that we know almost nothing about how it grows or how to cure it. You can have all the best experts, the best hospitals and even unlimited resources and still be lost without a cure. There is no way to learn, travel or buy your way out of a terminal disease. Determination, faith and a little bit of chance are your best hope. Stage 5 saw us attempting to preserve Elena's life. We bought concrete handprint pavers, had her paint walls and kept every last scrap of paper that she scribbled on. But now, at day 135, we realize that these stages were both premature and irrelevant. Elena is still fighting every day and will continue to do so. She now is exceeding expectations, just as we had hoped she would. Stages end here and living begins.

The journal was started late one night and continues today late into the night. Interestingly, Elena started a diary of her own today from a journal she received in her Easter basket. I guess she figured that if I could write, she could draw. Not to be left out, Gracie started her own diary too. But instead of calling it her diary, she calls it her "diarrhea." Tonight at dinner, she proudly announced that after she finished her green beans, she would need to "start her diarrhea." So much for the sanctity of the situation. Once again, Gracie teaches us to live in humor and with a smile. And that's just what we plan to do. Every day starting now is a gift.

Day 138—APRIL 15

A good day is relative, and while they certainly don't measure up to the good days of last year, our perspective and appreciation have changed. Today was a good day. For the first time in a while, we had the entire Sunday to ourselves. This meant a trip to the museum, where the girls played for hours and returned home quite sleepy.

I agreed with Gracie and decided that I would take a little nap on the couch. Thirty minutes later, Elena succumbed to her exhaustion and made her way to the couch to join me. This was the best part of my day. For the first two years of her life, napping with Dad was a Sunday tradition. During the fall and winter, we'd turn on the football game and I'd lie on the sectional with her in my arm.

Now, four years later, napping with Dad is still a Sunday tradition. And when Mom came home from errands two hours later, she found us lying on the couch, Elena's head resting on my shoulder, both of us wide awake but very comfortable. Who can sleep when you're afraid of missing a moment of this quality time? Either way, with Gracie awake and Mom pushing us to leave for the next errand, Elena and I pledged to continue our Sunday tradition next week too.

Day 139—APRIL 16

Tonight we moved the girls to Elena's room to sleep. With the removal of joists below Gracie's floor during the reconstruction of our house, we thought it best to move them for the night. But instead of Elena sleeping in her bed with Gracie tucked in on the floor mattress, Elena asked to instead sleep on the floor closer to the ground for fear she would fall out. Any other time, Gracie would have leapt at the opportunity to sleep in the "big kid" bed. But this time, the girl who anxiously awaits any chance of bunking her beds and getting the top bunk tiptoed downstairs to consult Mom and Dad. After all, why did she have to sleep in the "big kid" bed? "When is Elena going to get better?" Some questions were impossible to answer; others didn't make sense. "Will the house be finished when Elena gets better? I want presents just like Elena." Either way, we realized that Gracie had noticed.

Today it was her turn to be the big sister. Proudly, Brooke and I have seen Gracie not only express love for her sister, but grow far beyond her years. In pictures, Gracie now wraps her arms around her sister and pulls her close, just as Elena had done for the past four years. When we get in the car, Gracie now leans over to buckle Elena's seat belt and make sure she is comfortable before we leave the driveway. When they brush their teeth, Gracie now helps Elena open the toothpaste and apply it to her toothbrush. Tonight she tucked Elena into bed and gave her a kiss on the cheek. In all ways, she has not only assumed Elena's role as the big sister, but has been there to help her "bestest friend in the whole world."

Somehow I know this is not the last time we will need to console Gracie, nor will it be the last time she will fail to understand the changes in her sister. What I do know is that Gracie will never disappoint us or her "Lena."

Day 145—APRIL 22

I miss those warm sleepless nights. Not that we don't have our share of sleepless nights now, but then it was different. We'd go to bed around 9:30 P.M. and listen to sounds of the neighborhood children laughing and playing tag in the backyards of local homes. Of course at the time we'd curse the screaming and kick-the-can calls, wondering what kind of parents would let their children play outside after dark on a school night. After all, some of us have to be up at 4:30 A.M. But soon I would realize that my girls would also grow up and torment our neighbors with games of tag and screaming long after nightfall, just not on school nights. So I'd flip over, cover my ears and promptly go to sleep.

Tonight I hear the familiar screams and games being played outside our open windows. Somehow, though, this time it is different. At a time when I should be hearing my girls playing outside, I only hear their friends. With Elena sick, there will be no late nights, no games of tag and no screams.

Tonight after putting the girls to bed, Brooke and I sat on the top step of the stairway and listened—listened to the silence and listened to the breeze blowing through our windows. It was in that breeze that we heard the first whisper from Gracie to Elena. She had a plan: Elena will press the doorbell hanging from her headboard and make up something ridiculous. Never mind that we installed the doorbell for emergencies and bathroom runs; the girls use it as their personal call button.

Elena pressed the button and I entered the room, pretending to be worried, only to find that Elena wished to have toast in the morning. I feigned frustration and left the room. The doorbell rang again. This time she wanted to make sure I put all the money back in her bank that we had used for physical therapy that morning. I told her that I had, and I asked her to use the doorbell only for emergencies. She and Gracie giggled. And by the time I closed the door, I heard the doorbell once more. I waited. It rang again. I waited. It rang again. As I opened the door this time, they both burst into laughter; Dad was wrapped around their fingers and they knew it. Elena had no reason for ringing it this time; she just wanted to see my face as I raced in and started to tickle them.

Twenty minutes later, we were still playing the doorbell game, only this time they would ring the doorbell and then hide under the sheets. Too bad I still knew where they were. And tonight, if only for half an hour, it was our house making all the noise in the neighborhood. There were screams, giggles and even an occasional doorbell. Bedtime may be a little late tonight.

Day 146—APRIL 23

The leap from age six to thirteen occurs much sooner than you think. While her body and mind are still in kindergarten, her attitude today was pure teenager. She ignored adults, cut in front of her classmates in line and even engaged in a bit of back talk. Ignoring adults, I expected. When her music teacher came in to visit at recess, I justified the behavior by explaining that she was embarrassed about her voice. And while this has been true in the past, after hearing her talking to her classmates at snack time, I knew she was getting used to the sound of her voice. Suffice it to say, after her teacher left, we spent the remainder of the recess discussing how being sick does not excuse rudeness. Even at this, she did not make eye contact. At least she heard it.

It's when I see this determination and stubbornness that I begin to become hopeful that she will make it through this as the one-in-a-million child, the one who beat the impossible cancer. After all, if she can outlast me, why not a little disease? And while I know this is a distorted view, it's this strength that buoys our spirits. But then, optimism can be dangerous. As a parent, somewhere deep within, you prepare yourself for the worst. You protect yourself; you protect your heart. You look at her rebelling and find your mind wandering toward the future: her wedding, her children, your grandkids. Then you awake and realize it's still today and you're no further than you were two minutes ago. The fight is for today and it is one step at a time. Hope is what fuels you, but hope is also what discourages you. So you continue the day looking for hope but careful to not take it too far and fall into despair.

Elena is strong, stronger than I will ever be. If there is to be hope, it will be with her. In the meantime, it is our responsibility to support her, love her and teach her. Tomorrow we'll start with manners first.

Day 149—APRIL 26

I've heard them all. "God has a plan, though we may not understand it." "God works miracles." "God only burdens those he knows can handle it." From friends and family, they come without offense and are meant to comfort. I know this, but somewhere deep down I can't help but question.

Right or wrong, I've always found religion and God in my family. For me, I've never looked to the church, statues or the Bible for guidance. Instead, it is in the faces of my family that I've always found comfort and solace. These were the true gifts in life and somehow I always envisioned that I could seek virtue through my actions and commitment to my family. When Elena and Gracie were born, I knew that this was my mission. This was God's plan and I didn't need a sermon to tell me so. Today I find myself questioning not only my faith, but also God's plan. I look at Elena and I have a hard time believing that this is part of a "plan." After all, how can you find purpose in the loss of one of the most innocent of lives? She is my angel.

Tonight as the storms passed overhead and I kissed the girls for the final time before bed, I stood on the front porch searching for meaning. I looked to the east, to the south, to the north and finally to the west. I looked across the horizon and to the approaching storm front. Still, I could not find what I was looking for. To me, God is still in the faces of my children, as I think He will always be. No sky, church or priest can tell me otherwise. Still the storm keeps looming overhead, while I stand alone questioning. In two days we'll know more as we travel once again to Memphis for a checkup. I fear it will be too much for me to handle.

Day 152—APRIL 29

We disagree. As I write this Brooke is downstairs with Gracie in the Memphis hotel lobby while I sit with Elena in the room. To Elena it's just another fight among many we've had lately. Hopefully she'll never understand what we're arguing about. Brooke wants to keep trying. She tells me it isn't progression, that the drugs Elena takes will work and we just have to give it time. I disagree. She's getting worse, the drugs are wasting time and we need to switch. To what I don't know; it seems that no one does. Still, there's got to be something better.

Worse yet, her doctors also disagree. And in the balance hangs my daughter's life.

It's our worst argument ever, but this time it matters. Just like every other husband and wife, we disagree. Mostly it's about finances, a stupid comment or work. Then in an hour or two we either give up or forget what we were arguing about in the first place. But this time it's different. This time it's about Elena and I don't want to be right. Being right is an admission that we might have already lost and that we've wasted the last month when we could have been trying something new. Being right means that Elena's hope is reduced to weeks and not months. Being right means that we made the wrong choice. Being right means that we'll lose our daughter. I want nothing more than to be wrong. Still, I can't ignore the signs. The paralysis grows by the day. Each morning I see it in her face as she awakes and realizes she's still sick and not getting better. Slowly her eyes drop to her body and her smile fades. And I know that she's wondering what she lost overnight. Was it her vision, her hearing or maybe something simple like her big toe? She's smart enough to realize what's happening and I'm too close to ignore the signs. It's not getting better.

Today I asked the doctor about other options. Only after asking twice did he answer. The alternative is a treatment that it seems no one wants to recommend, at least not yet. It's untested and comes with a high risk of bleeding. He's not even sure if he can administer the drug with her in her current condition. And so we discuss side effects while my daughter is dying by our side. And I still don't agree. What's the side effect of doing nothing?

Brooke has a point. Without viable alternatives we should wait until the doctors agree. I just don't know if I'm that patient. There have to be other options—we have to do something. She'll never give up hope and I'll never compromise. And I don't know how it will end—either for us or for Elena.

So Brooke sits downstairs with Gracie while I sit with Elena while she sleeps.

Day 153—APRIL 30

I hate New York. I hate Cleveland even more. Nothing against the cities—personally I've never spent enough time in either to develop an opinion—but for today they symbolize something. You see, Elena listens to every conversation we have nowadays. When we say "MRI," her ears perk. When we say "bleeding," she turns to look. When we say "progression," she stops. Today we said "progression" quite a bit. Finally all the doctors agree: the tumor has grown and she is officially in progression. With an overall growth of over half a centimeter, the chemotherapy is no longer an option. In her case, it will provide no more hope and we must move quickly. But with pinhead bleeding, an established protocol is off the table. The options we had a month ago when her MRI showed no signs of bleeding are now nonexistent. Instead, thanks to the help of the hospital, we will pursue a new chemotherapy outside of trial and at our own risk, or rather Elena's. Unfortunately, this may also mean without the help of health insurance.

No one truly knows how this new treatment works or if it will work on diffuse gliomas, but when you have no other alternatives, nothing else matters. Together the hope is that it will provide the success that we once thought the previous chemotherapy would bring three months ago. However, with this treatment, bleeding is a serious concern. And with Elena listening in, we've started to refer to this bleeding risk as "going to New York." So when we say that she could have a very good chance of "going to New York," we must accept the risk before proceeding. Unfortunately, a "trip to New York" will most certainly result in a "trip to Cleveland," which means that she may not make it.

There, I've said it. And while I cringe at the callousness of these metaphors, with her in the same room as we continued conversations with her oncologist, I can't dare let her know the seriousness of the situation. As far as she is concerned, she will improve each and every day, despite the fact that for the last week, I've been struggling to find any improvement. Sadly, she may already know. Whereas before she would question every discussion we had with her doctors, she now sits in the corner motionless with her eyes locked on the floor. I know she is listening and I fear she even understands what we say when we talk about "going to Cleveland." She is smarter than I could ever know.

Tonight we go back home.

Day 156—MAY 3

She's hardly the artsy type. She loves numbers and details, doesn't wear eclectic glasses and has both ears, but somehow she's made it into the art museum right next to the likes of Picasso, Renoir and van Gogh. Okay, so I do know how she made it into the art museum, but to her, it is the ultimate wish. And although you may not notice her smile through the fog of a tripled steroid dose and the extreme exhaustion that accompanies a first dose of chemotherapy, trust me, this means the world to a six-year-old girl.

Today we took her painting to the museum to have it "installed." While we simply hung it on the wall of our living room, at the museum it would need to be "installed." There at the museum, Elena also had her first look at the gallery where her painting was to be displayed. Somehow, in the back of my mind, I envisioned her painting occupying a corner near the bathroom, where *Dogs Playing Pool* had been the previous masterpiece. But as we approached the gallery, we soon discovered that Elena's painting would take center stage in a room of giants. Picasso took the skinny wall by the door, while Elena's *I Love You* would reign supreme on the main wall flanked by masterpieces that otherwise could have had a gallery to themselves. And as if this was not enough, as we arrived, curators were desperately preparing the wall for Elena's picture with a fresh coat of paint and plaster. At home during our renovations, we'd be lucky if it even hung straight. I guess that's the difference between an installation and a plain old nail.

Since Elena's diagnosis, her artwork has taken on new meaning. Pictures that we'd otherwise toss are now priceless. Even scraps of paper that filled her school bag became testaments to her love. Now everything must be saved: every picture, every note and every card. Sometimes this is too much. In our desperation to save every memory, her room has become more of a shrine than a bedroom, forcing her to sleep in her sister's room for fear of the avalanche of stuffed animals, artwork and memorabilia. But how do you clean a room when you don't want to give up anything? You can't, so we spend our time rearranging, all the while convincing ourselves that it looks cleaner than when we started. One day I fear we'll need to add another wing to her

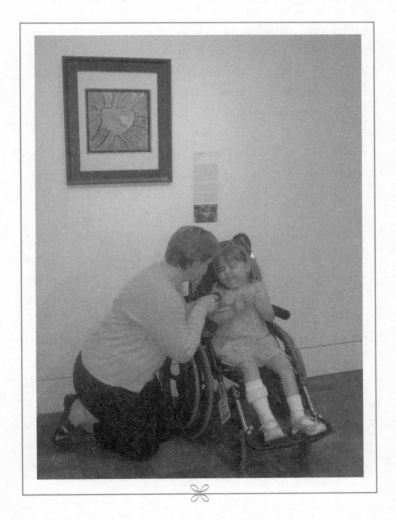

room. But then, I guess that is a good thing, as it will mean that she's still with us.

How she came to love art I still don't understand. Brooke hates the art museum and I can barely paint the walls of our house without making a mess. Yet with the ease of a trained professional, Elena refers to van Gogh and Picasso as if they were personal friends from school. Maybe they are and maybe this is just the result of a simple art class. Still I wonder if the other kindergarteners take these lessons as seriously as Elena does. Books of art line her shelves and a trip to the art museum is an occasion to be celebrated. And this time it's no different. Regardless, we'll continue to archive her pictures and she'll continue to paint. Without a voice and even a right hand, this is how Elena communicates with us and how she shows us her love. I guess that's why the title *I Love You* is so appropriate. Simple, plain and exactly Elena.

For Brooke and me, Elena's painting represents more than just a heart. It represents her ability to illuminate a disease that destroys so many young lives. It represents the vibrant colors and emotions that define our daughter. It represents her view of the world at this young age. Tears or not, we know that she appreciates the support and the one chance for her to see her painting at the art museum next to "her Pablo."

In the end, the painting was beautiful. Not because it was the best in the class, for I doubt it was. And not even because it hung in an art museum. It was beautiful because it symbolizes everything we love about our daughter—the power to illuminate and the willingness to share—all while being smaller and more reserved than the paintings around it. I love you, Elena.

Day 157—MAY 4

So many people spend their whole lives focusing on issues that don't really matter. I only wish we still made the same mistake. Today I am so grateful to God for something very simple, a thank-you. Today was the long-awaited kindergarten field trip to the zoo. At the beginning of the week, I fretted over mentioning this event to Elena for fear that we would not return to Cincinnati in time to attend. This morning, we were dressed in record time and she even ate all her breakfast pretty quickly (less than an hour). We packed our bags and started out the door until Elena stopped me and feverishly made a sign I had never seen before. She desperately tried to say the words, but after four hours of sleep last night, my brain could not wrap itself around what she was trying to say to me. Finally she pointed to paper and she wrote out, "I wut to sho mi snak." To clarify to those parents not skilled in kindergarten phonetic spelling, she was not asking for a Chinese snack, she wanted to take her new stuffed snake to show her friends.

I have no idea why, but my little girl dressed in a pretty pink dress had chosen a brown stuffed snake at her last visit to the hospital gift shop. Today she insisted on taking it to school. I think she was hoping that the kids would focus on the snake rather than the wheelchair the snake was coiled around. While it worked, I think it also helped that the kids were so preoccupied with the field trip. Her new wheels were low on their radar. Her mood was so improved that she even volunteered to say the Pledge of Allegiance over the intercom this morning. Elena didn't open her mouth the entire time, but she was smiling ear to ear as her three friends made up for her silence.

The rest of the day was a blur. We followed her classmates through the bears and monkeys. Elena requested that we visit the reptile house and she smiled at the irony as she showed her snake the other snakes. How I wish she could talk and tell me what hilarious joke was surely going through her head. We stuck with a small group of four girls from her class. As usual, they held doors and walked holding on to her armrests. Children are amazingly accepting, and her classmates have been able to make Elena feel more normal than we ever will be able to. After lunch we treated her friends to a carousel ride and after a quick picture, we left a little early.

As I drove home from the zoo, Elena was attempting to talk to me. Usually I can figure out what she says to me if I hear her and watch her lips. (Let's just say that this is a difficult feat while driving a car.) So at a stop light, I pulled down the rearview mirror and asked her what she was saying. She looked at me in the mirror, smiled and signed, "Thank you." My heart melted. Through all the nasty moodiness that the steroids cause, she was genuinely happy and I was so grateful I could find a way to bring that to her.

Day 159—MAY 6

I'm known as "Elena's dad." Nothing else matters after today and I'm okay with that. After having her artwork displayed at the art museum and her story carried on the front page of the newspaper, Elena has become a bit of a hero in her own right. Hopefully the most that I can ever aspire to be known as is "Elena and Gracie's dad."

Elena's recovery continued today in a manner all her own.

The leg is still weak and the right hand still hangs lifeless by her side, but her appetite has returned and her voice is improving. Not that she's giving up sign language any time soon. She's still busy teaching us two to three new signs a day. Where she learns it from we have no idea, but a quick check of the Internet confirms our suspicions: she's a sign language savant. This is her new voice and sometimes I wonder if she'll ever give it up.

As I kiss her good night, I try to remember the sound of

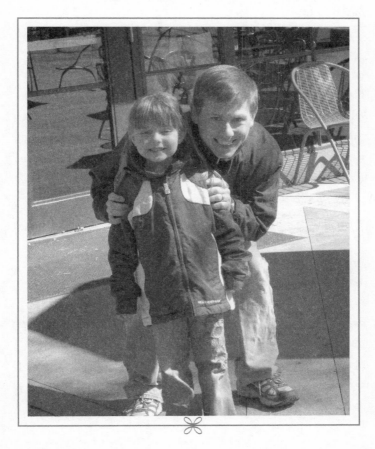

her voice. These are the moments that a camera doesn't capture. There's the smile, the face and the memories, but the voice is forgotten. Funny how you can forget something so important so quickly. For six years it was the sound of her voice that welcomed me home from work, the sound of her voice that begged to go higher on the backyard swing and the voice that wished me good night. Now it is the sound I can't remember.

Day 161—MAY 8

Every night when I clean out Elena's school folder, I pull out no fewer than two notes from Elena saying, "I love you Mom Dad Grace." I find the phrase on the back of her worksheets and on meticulously cut hearts. Just recently with her increased reliance on Mom and Dad to do the simplest of tasks, she has become ever more thankful for our help. Each time she makes the sign for "potty" and I approach to lift her, she smiles sheepishly. When she requests a toy or her fifth course of her meal, she signs, "I love you." When I carry her to the car for school, I get endless kisses as a thank-you.

Elena has always been an independent girl, and now she is painfully aware of her inability to control anything in her life. Yet, despite being miserable in knowing that she needs assistance to simply play with a toy, she is always quick to show us her appreciation. Just today Elena was sitting behind Keith as he talked to me about her upcoming medical appointment. Elena secretly signed, "I love you," with a broad smile on her face and I returned the smile just as brightly. Keith looked at Elena and back at me, questioning what we were smiling about. Elena simply smiled back

at him and rolled her eyes toward the ceiling, happy to find a way
to tease Daddy.

Day 163—MAY 10

Elena is an author. And at two books a day, I think she'll soon eclipse J. K. Rowling. Still, Elena's kindergarten teacher thinks that Elena should write less nonfiction and more fiction and instructional books. Apparently kindergarteners now need a writing portfolio. A lot has changed since my kindergarten, when I scribbled a crayon line on a piece of construction paper and went back to eating paste. Of course, I guess all that paste may also be why I never wrote prose. Still, I wonder if a journalistic exposé will be next.

Either way, Elena was determined to cure this problem and she started this morning at breakfast. The title: *How to Be a Kindergartener.* It was for her sister. You see, Brooke and I recently discovered that Gracie is fifteen days shy of the kindergarten cutoff for next year. And while we've always prided ourselves on not being overly aggressive parents, pushing advancement for the sake of advancement, we've decided that Gracie is ready. I think Elena agrees.

So somewhere in the midst of our discussions, Elena figured out that Gracie would be attending kindergarten and she decided that this should become the subject of her instructional manual. Then, armed with this new textbook, she decided she would coach Gracie on the finer points of kindergarten etiquette. So starting on the first page with a heart, she decided to show her the ropes. First, she determined that Gracie would need to learn to sit on the rug. This is where every good kindergartener must begin the day, sitting cross-legged and quiet as they begin to share. As if to help illustrate her point, she continued with a detailed drawing of the carpet squares, complete with marking to signify Gracie's place at the front of the room (do you think Elena knows something about Gracie's personality that we don't?).

On page two, Elena figured that Gracie would need a floor plan to better understand the elementary school campus. There are three areas at school: the top, the blacktop and the lower playground. This is where recess is held, and she went to great effort to not only list the areas, but to also draw a diagram to help Gracie understand how they relate to each other.

Page three was blank. I guess we must have skipped a page. Maybe she just left it with the understanding that she would add to it later.

Page four was dedicated to the complex kindergarten schedule. You see, not only do you have to worry about sitting on the rug, but you also have to balance art, PE, "muizc" (music, for all you non-spellers) and "libre" (that's Spanish for "library").

Page five contained only the simplest of instructions: "be qiit in the cafuteryu," or "Be quiet in the cafeteria." I think all teachers would be proud of this lesson, although I expect they'd want quiet in more places than just the cafeteria.

Page six was the most important page. Even with her limited voice, this was a subject worthy of elaboration. Ten minutes later, she was still instructing Gracie. This one was about Razzle Dazzle, the all-important honorary status bestowed on only one special child per day. The responsibilities are endless, the privileges are coveted and the daily tributes are legendary. He or she is the line leader, the password chooser and the weather forecaster. Best of all, it comes around only once every twenty-one days (there are twenty-one children in her kindergarten class). Elena's lesson to Gracie was simple: you get to be Razzle Dazzle. Who knows, you might even get a song named after you . . .

> *Her name is Elena,*
> *She's like the sun,*
> *Her Razzle Dazzle has just begun.*
> *Razzle, dazzle, sparkle and shine,*
> *Razzle dazzle, sparkle and shine.*

And trust me, after the first time your child becomes Razzle Dazzle you *know* the song. Elena sang it all the way home.

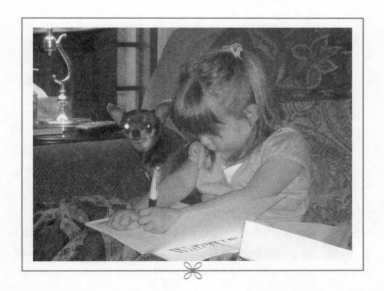

Page seven was simple. No words, just a picture of Gracie and all the friends she will make at school.

Page eight was blank. I guess she left more space to add to later.

Page nine was about calendars. Every good Razzle Dazzle girl needs to know how to read a calendar for news-and-weather time. Elena would later educate Gracie on the finer points of calendar function as she referred to her highly detailed diagram that continued on page ten.

Page eleven was all about attitude: "Smile Gracie." Apparently Mom and Dad's endless prompting for Elena to smile regardless of her steroid dosages had finally taken hold.

Page twelve was about Elena's favorite part of school, writing the nonfiction books that she loved. Now it was her turn to pass it on to Gracie. Writing, reading, word study, puzzles and math; the choices were endless.

Page thirteen was her tribute to her sister: "have a grat tim at knidrgrdni."

Page fourteen continued with a mission to "do gret weth ur tchr." Just like Elena, I have no doubt that Gracie will be the teacher's pet.

Pages fifteen and sixteen were all about the benefits of kindergarten. First she noted that in kindergarten you have poetry books. Then she noted the role of special activities like guests and programs.

Pages seventeen and eighteen summarized Elena's experience in kindergarten with "we have los uv fun" and "knidrdnd is los uv fun." And by the time she finished reading, Gracie was already packing her schoolbag. For Elena, kindergarten is fun and she couldn't imagine anywhere else she'd rather be. To her it represents new experiences, new friends and a routine that she so desperately needs right now. She always wants to be a teacher and now she gets to be a mentor. Good thing Gracie is a fast learner.

Day 165—MAY 12

For Mother's Day, the girls gave Brooke tomatoes. Well, not exactly tomatoes, but tomato plants. So there we were, parading around the yard in our muddy gym shoes, with muddy socks, wiping our muddy brows and doing our best to find some plant-able clay. Real quality time.

It occurs to me that I have never really grasped the meaning of the Mother's Day holiday. After all, for Mother's Day, Brooke asked for tomatoes, and she *hates* tomatoes. So why would she want tomatoes? Simple: it was for the girls. My mother has a tomato plant at her house and the girls love picking the ripe tomatoes directly off of the vine and popping them in their mouths. Sometimes they'd actually sit on the porch waiting for the tomatoes to turn red just so they could eat them. Now of course that never happened, so occasionally they'd pop a green one. This was more often the case with Gracie; she never had patience. Elena, on the other hand, would wait patiently until it was just perfect, but with Gracie around, her tomato selection would be limited.

On a day when we honor our mothers by rewarding them with any whim they can imagine, Brooke can think only of her girls first. No pedicure, no facial; for Brooke it is enough to simply ask for a planter for the one food that she hates the most. This was when I realized how lucky we are. Not only does Brooke think of her daughters first, but she also knows that her husband barely gets anything right, so she even sends him reminders. How lucky we all are. No card, no breakfast in bed, just tomatoes.

Day 166—MAY 13

Today was the day for the Eiffel Tower. And if you've been following Elena's wish list, you know that this was *the* wish— well, other than the chili parlor. A hundred and sixty-six days ago, after receiving the news that Elena might only live for a hundred and thirty-six days, she and I stayed up all night at the hospital and talked about what she wanted to do when we left. Little did she know what this list was about or that I would be committed to making it all come true.

On that list was wish number two: a visit to the Eiffel Tower. But not the Eiffel Tower in Paris; instead, the Eiffel Tower at the local amusement park just north of our house. Having driven by it on the way to Brooke's parents' house for more than six years, Elena always wondered what it would be like to look out from the top. So today, with clear skies and a perfect 72 degrees, we finally went to the park to climb the tower. Of course, it didn't hurt that the park staff had heard of Elena's wish and donated tickets for the cause.

About an hour into our visit and after overcoming Gracie's overwhelming desire to ride some rides, we finally boarded the elevator to the top and perched Elena's wheelchair next to the glass wall as we ascended the 354-foot tower. But with her new-found fear of heights, which we acquired somewhere during the disease, she was decidedly less than excited and wanted to be at least five feet from any overlook. That limited her appreciation to mostly the east, west, north and south horizons, but the effect was the same.

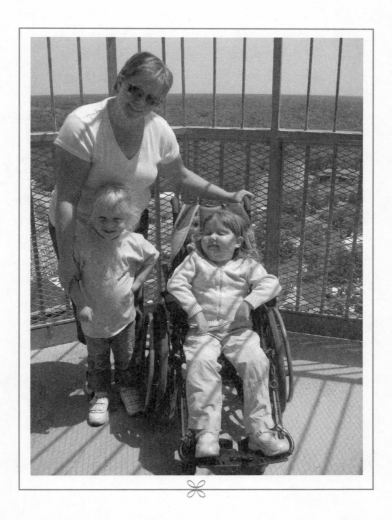

For Brooke and me, the occasion symbolized a triumph over the 135-day time frame. To Elena, she just kept looking for her kindergarten teacher's house (apparently at school, her teacher had told her that she could see her house and dogs from the tower). We never found the house with the two dogs in the backyard, but we did at least get a picture to remember. Soon it was time to board the elevator again, this time with our backs to the glass wall of the elevator, and continue our visit to the park.

While she had made tremendous progress in the last two to three days, today I noticed a decline. The finger no longer moved as it had previously, the right foot dragged once again, her speech was slurred and her breathing was labored. In my head I told myself that it was allergies, lack of sleep or even the sun. Never wanting to admit that it might be something else, I looked for excuses and even tried to ignore the signs. With so many positives in the past week, neither Brooke nor I wanted to see her this way. And while we may be overanxious, tomorrow will tell the true story. Either it was sleep and sun, or it was the tumor. Alone, none of her symptoms mandate further action, but collectively they cause us concern as we prepare for bed tonight. And still, as if in denial, Brooke and I have not discussed the symptoms that I'm sure we both have noticed. Today was a good day and I don't think either of us wanted to lose that feeling.

Day 168—MAY 15

A wise lady, who also has a child with DIPG, once told me, "Never look at a day and think it is a bad day, because this may be better than tomorrow, so just thank God that you have the day at all." I can't tell you how many times this has gotten me through a day. Every day we believe that we are doing our best. That our efforts are stretched to their limits and that we can do no more. The goals and struggles we endure today are the most we will ever carry. That someday it will get easier, but it never does. What we believe today to be impossible will be inconsequential tomorrow. And so it continues.

It is called a survivor mentality. And for those who accept this responsibility, life is both a burden and a pleasure at all times, particularly with our experience with Elena. I have come to understand what being a survivor means. It is a title bestowed on those who see a glimmer of light in a hall of darkness. It is a person who has no doubts, no fear and only confidence, who at times seems irrational. It is a person who believes that he or she alone can find the solution, and that at the right moment, it will become evident. It is a confidence that exudes optimism hand in hand with faith.

I often wonder if we have what it takes to be survivors. Could we stand alone on a deserted island secure in the fact that we would find our way home? Or would we be relegated to scanning the horizon for a hope of being rescued? And would we then feel the constraints of pressures for which we had no solutions? No food, no shelter and isolation. Would this be too much? Would we think it could get no worse, only to discover that it did?

Being a survivor must be more than just an ability to find solutions; it must also be an ability to cope. Suddenly I understand what it means and I wonder if we are up for the challenge. I have no doubt that Elena is. At a time when she is at her worst and seemingly unable to accept any other burden, she still takes the time to be a sister to Gracie. And through it all, she helps her prepare for kindergarten, get ready for bed and even brush her teeth. For her, being a survivor is also about being human.

Some days, as I look across the table at her laboring to breathe or struggling to drink from a straw, I wonder how much more I can take. Would it be better to just have calm, regardless of the outcome? Or is life about more than being comfortable? Somehow I know the answer, although I ask it daily.

Life is about the struggle, the passion and the love that we share for our children. Still, I'm struck by the fact that somehow I think I'm the one struggling when it truly has nothing to do with me. This is Elena's fight and I am merely a spectator placed here to support and love. She is the true fighter and the true survivor. Ultimately Brooke, Gracie and I are left to embrace Elena and make her stronger daily. We do not have cancer, we do not experience paralysis and we do not have to face this terminal battle. Elena does, alone. And when she succeeds, our family will be one. If she fails, we will be lost and left to cope, as survivors. Life is about the battle and belongs to survivors.

Day 170—MAY 17

They say to not expect too much out of the first days after chemo. She may have diarrhea, she probably will have nausea and she will be exhausted. If Elena can give attitude to her parents, she can definitely be defiant to those doctors, and she certainly was. I let Elena sleep in this morning. For me, that only lasted until 7:30, when I needed to see her face. Now there is no thought that escapes my mind as I open that door. Today I crept into her room and found her staring at the ceiling, and I held my breath. But instead of heavy breathing or groaning about her right side not working, she simply turned her head to me with a huge smile. My heart soared; it didn't just make me feel good, it made me float on air.

Day 173—MAY 20

Exhaustion has set in. I've experienced physical fatigue many times before. I've been simply tired, lacking my normal sleep. But exhaustion is a completely different matter. I awake every morning too tired to sleep, realizing that I haven't had a dream in months. I get dressed only to realize halfway through the process that I've put on two different shoes and I'm not quite fully awake. I drive across town but can't remember what route I took. I sit down to eat and can't bring myself to eat even though I'm hungry. Or worse, I eat just to eat regardless of the fact that I'm already full. I've resolved myself to writing lists throughout the day in order to keep track of my schedule, only to later lose the lists. I find myself struggling to remember names of people that

I've known for years. And in my mind there is only one thought, every hour of the day: Elena.

I often wonder if Elena experiences this as well. Fatigue is certain; we see the effects of chemotherapy on her face and in the number of naps she takes every day. Exhaustion is another thing. Today I think we saw it for the first time. We did our best to counteract it with aggressive physical therapy and an optimistic outlook, but the lines on her face tell a different story. After all, lines don't belong on a six-year-old's face. I could tell in the way she dragged her foot more while walking today despite being able to flex it during therapy more than ever before. I could tell in her hand as she let it slump over the armrest of her wheelchair no more than an hour after using it to hold down the corner of the prints she signed in preparation for the art show. And despite our best intentions, I watched as she gave up and went to sleep on the couch. She never truly naps during the day.

We ask her what she is thinking, believing somehow that by knowing her thoughts we will be able to give her peace. It's a dangerous risk, and if she asks the one question we hope she won't, we'll have to lie. So we hold our breath and ask. Today she told us that she loved watching everyone buy her painting and that it made her happy to see it at the art show. Thankfully today the answer was a good thing. Still, her exhaustion as well as ours is taking its toll. Sadly, there is no way out and no end, or at least not one we want.

Day 174—MAY 21

Today we started small. Five years ago, she learned to walk by first learning to crawl, so we thought this was the best way to start. The wheelchair became a method of transportation and nothing else. If she wanted to sit at the table, she had to walk to the chair and sit down. If she wanted to draw and make a craft, she would do so on the floor. And when her pen was out of reach, she would have to crawl to get it. But when you've been in a wheelchair for the past month and a half, even the simplest activities become a challenge. A five-foot crawl to get a bead took ten minutes and involved falling to her belly more times than you can imagine. Still, by the end of the day, she realized that slow and steady movements were better than larger ones and when you stop crying you really can concentrate better.

What came naturally once must now be learned again.

On a side note, the next time you see Elena, ask her about Earl the Squirrel. It seems that at breakfast Elena made a bet with Mom that even the squirrel sitting outside on the retaining wall wouldn't eat her medicine. Mom held the moral high ground and put $5 on it. Tonight the medicine still sits on the wall and the squirrel is nowhere in sight. Tomorrow, either Elena will be $5 richer or you'll soon see a squirrel roaming our street with a bad attitude. Looks like Mom is going to lose again.

Day 176—MAY 23

One peanut butter and jelly sandwich, a cookie and chocolate milk. Sometimes a strawberry on those days when the steroid hunger sets in. Elena loves the picnics in the backyard. The breeze is cool, the grass is warm and the respite from the living room couch is always appreciated. This is the beginning of Wednesdays with Dad.

Sometimes we hear the hawk from above as she builds a nest in the oak tree overhead. Other times we can barely hear each other over the pounding of hammers and the scream of circular saws as the carpenters build the untimely addition on the back of the house. At one point, it seemed like a good idea, but now, after her diagnosis, it is nothing more than a distraction that we don't need. Still we move on, only this time reworking the plans to accommodate a first-floor bedroom and a handicapped-accessible bathroom just for Elena.

I ask her over lunch what color she wants to paint her new bedroom. She just shrugs. Maybe pink, I suggest. She looks away. We sit in silence. Somehow I think she knows more than I want her to. The house will be finished in October but her disease tells us to expect no longer than July. It is June. Somehow I doubt she will ever be able to decorate her new room.

We try to talk about something else, but small talk is all about the future. Questions like where she wants to go on vacation, "Are you looking forward to school?" and "What do you want for your birthday?" all seem frivolous. I think even she knows that she'll never make it that far. So we sit in silence.

We give these children gifts and vacations when we can't give them hope and a cure. And they know the difference. I believe that Elena does. I can see it now in her smile and in the pictures she draws. The themes are of love, but also finality. "I love you Mom, Dad and Grace," she writes, as if she'll never see us again.

After the picnic, we lie on our backs and look at the clouds, her head on my arm. We exchange no words, just a passing glance and silence. I love you too, Elena.

Day 178—MAY 25

How does cancer affect a child? How does it affect my child—aside from the clinical effects? Over the past two weeks, I've started to notice changes in Elena that I fear will never heal. Where there was once a child, there is now an adult. Where there was once innocence, there is now cynicism. Where there was once a smile, there is now scorn. The moments are fleeting but becoming more and more dominant over a six-year-old's carefree manner. Now I wonder if we will ever be able to bring back the child in her.

To question her future attitude is to assume there will be a cure. That is the good thing. And maybe the loss of a childhood will be the only thing we have to fear if the cancer goes away. That, by itself, is a leap of faith. But as she starts to recover again for the third time, we are back at the top of the hill with a view of the horizon and suddenly we start to question future prospects. At the bottom, you can only see the ground. So tonight as I washed her hair and put her to bed, I found myself searching for the girl I once knew. But in her eyes, all I see is emptiness and suspicion. After being poked and prodded, cut and bled, stretched and poisoned, she no longer can feign innocence. She is more of an adult than I will ever be.

Cancer or any terminal illness makes martyrs out of heroes and hollows souls out of survivors. Bringing innocence back will be impossible. No candy or flowers will allow her to forget this struggle; it is part of her life and part of her future forever. Still, it is the best that I can hope for, for survival is the only objective.

As a parent, you also begin to wonder how far to push. If this is not the cure, do we go beyond experimental and verge on improbable? And at what point should we give up? Can survival be worse than death? Right now, survival is our goal, and I will never be able to answer that question until it occurs. I pray to never see that day.

Day 181—MAY 28

In my family, you know you've made it when you get posted on the back of the bathroom door. The television stations pick up anything, the newspaper may fill space, Nobel Prizes are commonplace and even the Pope can recklessly choose a saint, but being featured on the back of my grandfather's bathroom door is a legendary honor. Why the bathroom door? Why not the kitchen bulletin board or the living room shelf? Who knows, but the back of the bathroom door has always been a place to feature the "movers and shakers" of the family. There you'll find a newspaper picture of my great-aunt and great-uncle as they participated in a breast cancer cure walk, an article on a relative who earned a "teacher of the year" award and a newspaper picture of my sister combing the tail of a horse before a show. These are the heroes of my family and these are the ones who will be honored for all of eternity on the back of the bathroom door. As a child, I could only wish to be that lucky.

Tonight, I have been informed by my grandfather that Elena has taken her rightful position as a bathroom-door honoree. Now we know that she has truly touched lives. Effective last week, her newspaper article and *I Love You* masterpiece will grace all who seek respite with the gods of indoor plumbing. Forever to enhance the color scheme and decorating of a bathroom ripped from the seventies, Elena's brilliant colors and shades of blue and pink will forever call out to visitors of my grandfather's bathroom to seek the betterment of themselves. And now, her impact will increase tenfold, mostly just because of the size of my family.

Kidding aside, the bathroom door represents something. It represents an achievement and the selfless impression that she continues to leave on my family. And while it may not measure up to a debut at the art museum among the likes of van Gogh and Picasso, a front-page story in the newspaper or even being the featured artist at the local art show, it is the one recognition that means the most because it is from her family.

On June 1 Elena will be honored by the city with a proclamation declaring it "Elena Desserich Day" for her impact on the city and its residents. Never before did I figure my daughter would have this much impact or be appreciated by so many. And in the beginning, I didn't even know what a proclamation was. But after reading the text that the city manager sent to me late last week, I now understand its significance. Even without the proclamation, we knew that we were the parents of two very special girls.

This Friday, when it is presented, I have no doubt that Elena will be impressed and honored. And if we're lucky, she might even smile through the steroids as she is given a copy of the proclamation complete with a large blue ribbon. They tell me that it might eventually hang with a copy of her picture at the local recreational center lobby for all to see and appreciate. To Brooke and me, this is more than we could ever hope for. Elena, on the other hand, would be perfectly happy if it were to only hang on the back of the bathroom door.

Day 182—MAY 29

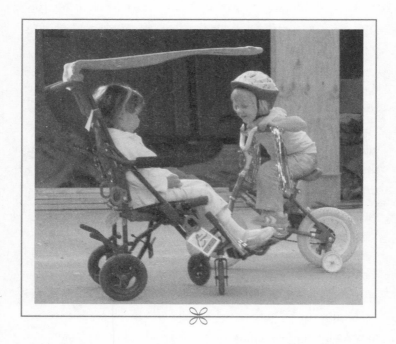

Gracie needs us now more than ever. But instead of playing with her on the swing, both Brooke and I spent the afternoon with Elena in the house. The weather has warmed and we should be outside with both girls enjoying the playhouse, pushing them on the swings and teaching them how to ride their bikes on the apron, but Elena can barely eat, let alone swing. So we sit inside watching Gracie through the window as she plays alone.

Increasingly I find myself having to choose and lately it's been Elena that I've spent time with. We know that her days are now limited, although we rarely discuss it, so we do our best to comfort her and love her. But by doing so, it is Gracie who loses. She loses her mom and dad, she loses the joy of a four-year-old's summer afternoons and she will ultimately lose her sister. And there is nothing we can do to prevent it. Brooke and I try to take turns, both knowing that the time we spend with Gracie will be time we spend wishing we were with Elena. So we choose between moments we'll regret and memories we will cherish.

In the end, Gracie's milestones are no less important than Elena's. But when a life is compressed into six short years, every second seems like a day. Gracie's moments will live on tomorrow—at least that's what we tell ourselves. Still, how do you trade one child for another? I hope Gracie understands—I'm counting on it.

So Gracie swings alone just for today. I fear this will not be the last time. And if we lose Elena will we find ourselves regretting the time we lost with Gracie? Is it any less precious? I don't know the answer. So we choose. Gracie swings alone while we cuddle with Elena on the couch.

Day 184—MAY 31

I have recently found it impossible to look at pictures. As the end of the school year approaches, we start to get sentimental.

I wish I was like every other parent, busily thinking ahead to summer camps and playdates, but instead of looking forward, I find myself looking back.

We picked up Elena's yearbook today. Prominently on several pages, Elena's bright smile and those big beautiful eyes that we knew would melt every boy's heart made her picture stand out. I couldn't control my emotions as I flipped the page and saw Elena decked out in her Indian headdress from their Thanksgiving lunch. That was the last day of innocence. The last carefree day. The last day of school before we whisked her away to endure endless days of doctors and treatments. Through her already strained voice that day, she told me of the food they ate and things they did. She excitedly told me about why she chose to be an Indian rather than a Pilgrim. I miss how she got so excited about learning. I am sure she still gets excited about school, but she just doesn't show it much anymore.

I just stared at Elena's picture and thought how beautiful and young she looked. I never knew a disease could age a girl five years in five short months. I am not even referring to her newly bulging cheeks. I look into her eyes and my heart sinks as I see how tired they look, how "experienced" they appear. Gone is the innocent sparkle that you see in all the kindergarteners. She knows more about this world than any of those children will for years to come, the good and the bad.

Day 185—JUNE 1

Holy cow, she has a sign! Gracie was as surprised as I was as we drove home from work this afternoon. Prominently displayed on the community recreational center billboard for all to see was the message "Today Is Elena Desserich Day." They were serious about this proclamation thing.

The day began with an early wake-up call from Gracie at 4 A.M. It seems that "Lena Day," as she calls it, deserved as much anticipation as Christmas. Perhaps she might have been disappointed by the lack of presents or tree, but Gracie was content to jump out of bed and snuggle up to her sister and wish her a happy Elena Day. Elena barely budged. Still, Gracie patted her cheek with her hand, kissed her and offered Elena her coveted "low" (her satin pillowcase that she sleeps with every night) as comfort. And after seeing the affection she presented her sister with, I didn't quite mind the early awakening.

The official proclamation ceremony took place at 6 P.M., after a long day (and two naps for Elena) filled with school and

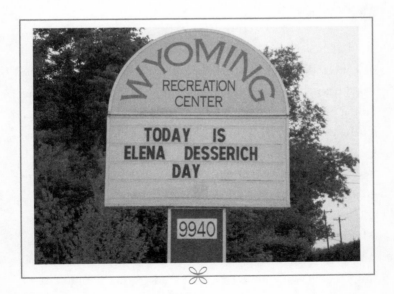

swimming. As part of the ceremony, Elena's painting would be officially mounted in the recreational center lobby alongside a notice declaring June 1 as Elena Desserich Day, as long as you live in the city. And there in our bathing suits, sunglasses and cover-ups, Elena was honored for her courage, bravery and inspiration. After a few "whereas"es, "therefore"s and "hearken"s were thrown in, it was made a legal and official proclamation for years to come.

Tonight, as Elena Desserich Day reaches twilight, her proclamation hangs on the wall of the recreational center as well as her bedroom for all to see. Still, in our hearts, tomorrow will always be more special than today, regardless of our newly certified holiday. Tomorrow brings promise, today brings hope. In the meantime, happy Elena Day! Holy cow, she has a sign!

Day 186—JUNE 2

Lately we've resorted to distraction to relieve stress. Instead of concentrating on her frustration with eating, we read the headlines in the local newspaper. When she can't even sit without falling over, we pick paint colors for the new addition. When her left hand fails, we try cleaning the house. Still, it never works. Headlines don't matter, colors are irrelevant and the house will never be clean again. Our thoughts are with Elena and the future no matter how hard we try to protect our sanity and ourselves.

It is the feeling of being out of control that hurts the most. After all, from the very beginning of life you are taught that if you do good, good will come to you. When you bring in the trash, you get an allowance. Good grades bring the promise of ice cream. But all along, control is the one thing that eludes you. Now we truly understand how little control we exert over our lives. As we look at Elena, we wonder to ourselves what we did wrong and how we can make it right. I'd like to believe that we've lived lives devoid of sin and to the benefit of others, but still I wonder if we could have done more.

It's a ridiculous notion; it doesn't happen for any reason at all to any particular person, but in the back of your mind you just can't shake it. You never will, regardless of how many times people tell you otherwise. Still, you want it to be true. Not because you want to find fault with yourself—guilt has nothing to do with it, no matter how many people make this assumption. Instead, you want it to be true because it will give your life meaning and grant you the faith that you crave.

After all, if life is about consequences and charity, you are back in control. You can excuse away tragedy on the basis of sin and perfect yourself in the pursuit of fortune. No longer will you fear life and question tomorrow, because life can be what you want it to be. And therefore time is endless and without true value. Good deeds mean more time.

In reality, it is better without control. For without control, time is the ultimate reconcilable factor. Good deeds are done not because of a promised fortune, but because they are the right things to do. And today is the only thing to be lived for. This is the lesson of Elena and the tragedy of a terminal illness. Sadly it is a lesson I wish we never would have to learn.

Even our journal is a distraction. On tough days, we turn to self-reflection, and on good days, we talk about how we spent our hours as a family. Today was not a good day. Elena couldn't stand, could hardly eat and couldn't even sit without falling over. And while they tell us that we need five days from treatment before drawing any conclusions, Brooke and I wonder how much longer we can wait. Tomorrow is the fifth day and we have not made any tangible improvement from the depths of Wednesday. So we watch TV, write a journal and look at paint swatches, all while thinking the one thought we still can't talk about.

Day 187—JUNE 3

The people at the gas station thought I was crazy. No, not just because I pulled up in an SUV when gas was at the highest price all year; that was about the only sane part of the fill-up. No, the looks came when I circled the car making faces and banging on the windows. Of course, what they couldn't see through the tinted windows was Gracie and Elena in the backseat smiling in delight at Dad's antics. You see, I'm not really crazy (at least not yet) so much as I'm looking for smiles. And in this game, it's all about the element of surprise and cheap visual gags.

I run from side to side, popping up in a different window each time with a different funny face. Then it's down again as I hunch over and run to the next window, careful to avoid tripping over the gas hose. This time I pop up over the hood and they see me through the front windshield. Next I bang on the rear, creating a shriek of surprise and laughter that only I can hear from outside the car. But after three trips, my back and legs scream out for relief, while inside the girls scream out for more. Too bad for me that I didn't buy the economy car—at least then the fill-up would be over. Instead, I'm only $40 into the visit and with an SUV this is only halfway. Now I'm left with the old tricks. I start with the stairway trick and then the elevator. Brooke rolls her eyes, but the girls want more. "Over here, Dad," yells Gracie as she points to her window. Apparently, the experience has special meaning if it is in her window. I oblige and move to the other side. Nearing the end, I finally hear the click of the gas pump and realize it's time to leave.

In the end, it's a smile and a laugh that I'm after. So next time you see me running around my car with arms flailing and banging on the windows, you'll know the girls are inside and I'm working for smiles. Stare all you want—then try it with your kids. Together we'll be the crazies at the pump.

Day 190—JUNE 6

You can feel the excitement in the air. It is the day before the last day of school. I am actually sad I wasn't able to make it to the last "real" day of school today. I hate tomorrow because I don't want school to end, and the progress to end, and the learning to end, and the purpose to end. Three months isn't an eternity anymore and I so desperately want to be standing there with her next year waiting for the school bell. I must have stared at the flyer to order school supplies for next year's class for about twenty minutes. I haven't wanted to fill out a form as badly as I did that one. Then I put down the form and got on the Internet in a desperate attempt to find just one survivor of DIPG. If only I could have hope.

Day 196—JUNE 12

Through her life, Elena has constantly been complimented on her stunning eyes and beautiful hair. To emphasize her long locks, she had the world's most eclectic variety of ponytail holders, clips and, of course, headbands. Headbands of every color and most of them sparkling with rhinestones or sequins. Elena never wore gaudy clothing, but she always knew the "bling" belonged in her hair. Just this year, she asked to start having the honor of brushing her hair before school and she meticulously made sure it was smooth and shiny before placing the chosen ornament of the day.

When we met with the doctors in the beginning, they warned of the possibility of thinning where the radiation beam would enter and exit her head. Even though we had slight thinning, she had such thick long hair she could easily hide it.

Elena's first chemo was a low-dose oral variety that did not cause hair loss. It was actually a bit weird to walk around the hospital with hair. Most days there were boxes of brightly colored knit caps at the front counter, where the kids could choose their daily accessory piece or do-rags made of fun material patterned with their favorite character. I still remember the time Elena, after noticing she was in the minority with hair, asked if she was going to lose her hair. After reassuring her she would not, she actually asked to pick one handmade hat that caught her eye.

Unfortunately this new chemo is much harsher and it is likely that she too will join the majority of her friends at the hospital wearing fun head coverings. Tonight, for the first time, I noticed a lot more hair in the brush. We asked her if she wanted to try a new hairstyle and she emphatically shook her head "no." We suggested *she just look at different styles to see if there was something she would like better and she just shrugged. I can't imagine how she would take losing her beautiful, long hair after she had such a tough time with the swelling in her face. Perhaps her thick hair will be forgiving and she will just have thinning. Either way, we will still have the most beautiful girl with big, bright eyes and the most lovable face. We will just have to expand our repertoire from hair ornaments to the fanciest head coverings anyone has ever seen.*

Day 198—JUNE 14

You desperately want to forget. These are not the memories that you want to keep when you remember your daughter. Instead, you want to remember her laughing as she chases her sister across the backyard or cradling a baby ever so gently in her arms. But today was not for memories. Today was about surviving. Still, the hours and moments are priceless and you hold them near.

Recovering from chemotherapy, Elena was unable to both eat and drink today without extreme difficulty. Every effort to bring a cup to her lips was met with gurgling and coughing, signaling us to stop for fear of causing pneumonia. The lips and teeth were equally resistant, clenched tightly together, preventing the passage of both spoon and straw. So for now, we concentrated on nutritional drinks delivered via dropper, one drop at a time. And when we weren't forcing food, she spent the balance of the day in her bed staring at the ceiling. I don't think she really slept, but to her it was an excuse to do nothing and she liked it. Thank goodness Grandma and Grandpa visited to take her out for a bit of swimming therapy or she would have spent the better part of the day getting to know her new favorite color—ceiling white. From what I hear, she kicked and floated the hour away. I wonder if they have ceiling white at the pool.

Somehow I never imagined that I'd feed my daughter with a dropper or that I would also succumb to the melancholy of her situation and allow her to stare off into the distance. It is not the memory I wish to remember and I never plan on repeating it. This was a day devoid of moral lesson and message. And for the first time I wondered what would happen if it were to end. Would it be fast or slow? How would we react? Would it be our fault? And in that instant, I also wondered if I could protect myself from her loss. Could I teach myself to ignore my feelings and fool myself into believing that it really didn't matter? But it was in asking that question that I found my answer. The very act of posing this question proved that it did matter and I couldn't stop caring or remembering. Still, today was not a day for memories or to be remembered. This thought process had to end. It did. Tomorrow we will make memories.

Day 199—JUNE 15

Comfort Care, Star Shine, Palliative Aid. Apparently there are endless names for the most dreaded step for cancer families. We started hospice today with great trepidation. Our doctor had hinted around about hospice for the last few weeks and urged us to meet with them, if simply just to talk. We fought it and insisted that we had it under control.

But grudgingly, we relented and signed up for hospice, if simply to prevent putting Elena through a night in the hospital. As soon as we made this decision, Elena instantly started drinking more and ate two bowls of ice cream and two pretzels. Miraculously, the mouth that couldn't find a way to open for Dad's mashed bananas was wide open to accept the frosted donut holes Grandma brought for breakfast. Also, on a positive note, her hand and foot were looser than they have been in weeks. Nevertheless, we went ahead with our plan to get her recovering faster.

This afternoon we met with the hospice team and our doctor. We talked about what we could do to make her comfortable and were amazed at what hospice actually offers. Only now do we realize why our doctor was so intent on us meeting with the team. I only wish I didn't fall into the trap of thinking hospice was giving up. I was excited to find out they even have a massage therapist for Elena. Somehow I know this will be her favorite.

They also spent the hour trying to teach two overly tired parents to remember the hundred-step process to get an IV bag connected. Then we spent the next hour giving them the hundred-step process to deal with Elena. We assured them they had the harder task at hand. They welcomed the opportunity to help Elena get back to her bullheaded and independent self. I suggested that if the nurse wanted to make friends quickly tomorrow morning that perhaps she needed to come with frosted donut holes. What started out as a dreaded conversation surprisingly gave me hope. This wasn't the beginning of the end; it was us accepting we may need some help from time to time.

Day 200—JUNE 16

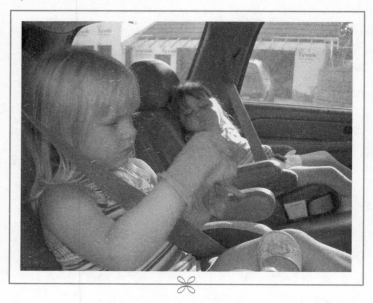

So much for being a police girl or teacher. Gracie informed us tonight that she's officially changed her career choice and this time it is final. Instead of "shooting bad guys" and teaching, she's made up her mind to be a doctor. But not just any doctor—she wants to be Elena's doctor. She wants to be a pediatric oncologist. After all, they get to wear blue gloves, use loud beeping machines and help kids. What could be better? And as she dangled her feet off the hospital bed, she whispered to Mom that the best part about being a doctor would be that she "could wear a big white coat." Time to start saving for college—and the coat.

So, donning her blue latex gloves that she deftly stole from the hospital and hid in her jean shorts pockets, she made up her mind. She was to be a pediatric oncologist and she had to "hurry up and grow up." After all, Elena needed her help and Gracie was determined to be her new doctor. "Doctor Gracie," as she now refers to herself. But in the car, Elena only shot her a stare of disdain. After all, wasn't this the girl who told us last week that she didn't want to feed the fish and we could flush them? Okay, so she'll have to learn some bedside manner along the way. In the meantime, she does have some nice blue gloves . . .

Day 201—JUNE 17

Lately, we've lived in fleeting moments. As the days grow, Elena's condition seems to be a contrast of alternatives. She has not recovered the way we hoped from the last chemotherapy treatment and now we consider what we had hoped to avoid. I know now what those before us have been through. Still, there are those signs that give us hope: the unintended smile before she coughs, the arm curled around my neck as I take her down the stairs, and the yawn. They say that her yawns are reflexive, but Brooke and I live for them. Whereas she can only open her mouth a quarter inch normally, with each yawn it opens completely. But what is most heartening is her voice, which reappears with every yawn to its fullest power and melody. Why, we have no idea, but with every yawn we hope that Elena's abilities will return and this will all be a distant memory. It isn't. Still, her yawns are moments to celebrate as we turn to remember the sound of her voice and the sweet song of innocence. We try to force a yawn, mimicking our own and feigning an exhaustion that we already have, but it is without result. So we are left to wait for the next occasion.

Try as we might, we are unable to remember Elena or her voice the way it was. So late at night we watch our thirty-second video clips from the hospital recorded on our digital camera. And while it still isn't her real voice, it's close enough for us to reminisce. Some days I wonder if we will forget the beauty of her face in this same way, or if we will just remember how it ended. I've been there before, as has virtually every other person who reads this—I just fear the thought.

I've also found that I've started to live between blinks. What is too painful to watch causes me to close my eyes, only to quickly open them for fear of missing a moment. I guess this is natural, but lately, as she falls to the floor, chokes on noodles or cries from exhaustion, I have spent more of the day with my eyes closed. Maybe once when I open them, she will suddenly be better. But this is only a dream. Somehow I do not think it will get better tomorrow.

Day 203—JUNE 19

I feel like I've run a marathon. For the past few days I have felt things I never wanted to feel, cried myself into a constant headache and probably tied my stomach into a knot a Boy Scout would be proud of. Keith and I have stayed up late each night trying to figure out how to make Elena eat so that she doesn't have to use a feeding tube. Tonight I started the two-hour process of trying to feed her for dinner. We tried to broaden our horizons and branch out from our constant yogurt consumption and try chicken and stars soup. After ten bites of this, she didn't want any more. I asked her if she wanted plain old milk, not the vitamin-packed milk we've been trying to force her to drink. She picked up the medicine cup and practically chugged it. She still coughed afterward, but it didn't stop Keith and me from standing dumbfounded.

Keith opened the cupboard to put away some food and Elena lifted a shaky finger. After playing twenty questions, we found out that she wanted Goldfish. She carefully chewed three Goldfish. We then opened the refrigerator and cupboard for her to choose what she wanted. Her dinner was three Goldfish, half a slice of cheese, a scoop of ice cream and, as a reward, a mouthful of whipped cream. So much for healthy—at least it isn't a feeding tube. Each "course" was carefully chewed and she coughed often, but it went down.

After Dad took Gracie up for bed, I asked Elena if she wanted more to eat. She shook her head no and pointed to her cheeks. I finally figured it out: she was afraid if she ate too much her cheeks would grow bigger. I told her she was beautiful and she shook her head "no" and pointed to her cheeks. We tried to explain that it was the steroids that caused the cheeks to swell and not the food, but she refused to believe us. If she only knew.

Day 204—JUNE 20

So far everything they've told us was wrong. They said she'd live three months beyond radiation or 135 days. We're on day 204. They told us that she'd make it maybe seven months. Next week she'll surpass that marker. They told us that after progression, we might have three weeks left. She's already made it nine weeks beyond that point. And now when we are told to prepare for the end after her recent bout with respiratory problems and contemplation of a feeding tube, we now find ourselves again taunting the inevitable. This morning she awoke, drank two glasses of milk and ate a full breakfast. By lunch she had crackers and cheese and was asking to go to the mall. Tonight the doctors tell us that they just don't know, and that's exactly what we want to hear.

The abnormal is our best hope. Normal is terminal, so abnormal must be life. Regardless of how it happens or the extent to which we can explain it, abnormal might also deliver a cure. This is how medical science is written—in small steps, abnor-

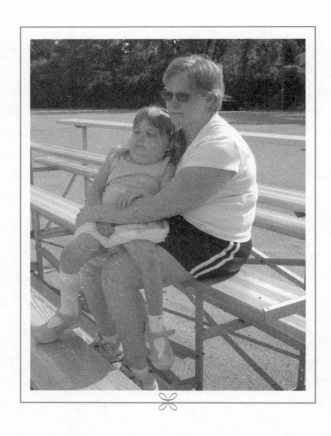

malities and trial and error. I truly believe that if we find a cure for DIPG, we will find a cure for *all* cancers. The solution lies in the most dismal cases and in the enduring spirit of our children.

In the end, pioneering medical science isn't so much about education or research—it's about courage and finding the ability to say, "I don't know." So tonight when her doctors took the time to come to our house during their free time, we found faith in their sincerity. And when they called Elena's condition "abnormal," both Brooke and I found comfort. And when they said, "I don't know," we cheered. Neither do we. Let's find out together. We're in very good hands.

Day 207—JUNE 23

Today we needed an excuse to pamper Elena. With the loss of the hair and the swelling in her cheeks, she needed all the indulgence we could offer. Gracie, ever the adventurous one, went first. Pink-and-red nails and Shirley Temple curls—what a sight! And knowing Gracie, nothing like you'd expect. No more tomboy—at least until the curls fall out. Elena, ever the timid soul, was fascinated with the stylist's wife's red highlights and finally decided to get some of her own. After three trips to the hairstylist for curls, braids and beehives, she needed something different—something that screamed rebel. Besides that, she just liked the color red. And I mean *red*! *Permanent coloring red!* So be it.

Mom and I were not about to say no to a girl who just spent the last seven months getting poked and prodded going in and out of hospitals from state to state. We'll hold the line at tattoos and piercings—at least for now. Somehow I think if she returns to the salon, a request for piercings and tattoos will soon follow.

Two hours later, Elena had her new style and cut, as well as a four-foot stuffed dog and a berry smoothie, all courtesy of the salon, which went out of its way to make Elena comfortable despite her ever-raging back pain. Maybe tattoos aren't all that bad—as long as they're not on my daughters. Either way, the trip was most certainly worth it and Elena loved showing off her new style. Maybe this will take her mind off her cheeks, if only for a little while.

Day 210—JUNE 26

We call them wild cards. And they usually happen at 2 A.M. She wakes up, pokes Mom and moans something unintelligible. We ask her if she wants to lie on her side. She shakes her head. We ask her if she wants to lie on her back. She shakes her head. We ask her if she wants the covers pulled over her arm. She moans again—this time we know she is saying no. We ask her if she wants another stuffed animal. She shakes her head. We ask her if her leg is hurting. She moans no. Now she's getting frustrated. We turn on the light, searching for any clue she might hold in her face as to what she wants. We ask her to say it again. This time we think she's telling us to "leave Grandma's coat off." We know this isn't it, but we don't dare repeat it for fear that she'll get angry and then the huffing and puffing will start. Time to wake up the house.

Before long, all the lights are on and it's an early morning game of charades. She tries to spell with her hands, but with her paralysis, all we can make out are E's and L's. Somehow this won't help. "Get the pad of paper!" Two minutes later, with paper in hand she draws a small U with a line over it. "Is this a picture or a vowel?" She just shakes her head. We ask if it is in her room. She shakes her head. We ask if it has something to do with her body. She moans no. That's when we ask the most important question of the night: "Does it have to do with tonight?" She shakes her head "no." Usually the routine goes like this and we continue guessing:

She wants to sleep on her side.

She wants to sleep on her back.

She wants to sleep on her other side.

She wants her hand brace.

She doesn't want her hand brace.

Her right leg has locked straight and needs a pillow.

She wants to put in her breakfast order.

She wants to tell you that she wants to sleep with Mom tomorrow night (never Dad).

She wants to tell you that she wants Mom to stay home with her tomorrow morning (never Dad, again).

She doesn't want therapy.

She wants her blanket adjusted.

She's just testing your reaction speed to the bell (she loves this one).

She's still asleep and lying on the bell.

She has to go to the bathroom.

Or a wild card . . .

Most of the time she asks for something simple like a drink or to go to the bathroom. Other times we get lucky and get it on the first or second try. But it's the wild cards that are the most difficult. This is when she wants to tell us something that has nothing to do with what she is doing at that time. Frequently it's just an observation and she doesn't want anything at all. She just wants to let us know about something she saw earlier that day. Other times, she wants to tell us about something she wants to do tomorrow or the next day. She'll tell us that she wants pink socks tomorrow or that she counted five flags on the way home from the hospital. Either way, it's nearly impossible to guess. Still, when she first lost her voice, we promised that as long as she never gave up, neither would we. Our reward: the largest and most precious smile you will ever see as she realizes that she can still communicate with us even through it all.

The speech therapist visited Elena today to help us improve our communication. Realizing that sign language will no longer work, we are turning to a picture book of symbols and words to help. So today we took pictures of nearly everything in the house that she could possibly ever want. We took pictures of her animals, her chair, her pillow and even her ice cream. Then we took pictures of her in bed—lying on her side, on her back and with the blanket over her body. The last group of pictures will go in a separate section of the book marked "Nighttime." Maybe now we can get a little more sleep. Last night alone, she woke up eight times. Seven of those times she wanted to be repositioned. One time was a wild card. That one wild card took longer to figure out than all of the seven combined.

If you're wondering, the wild card took us about thirty minutes to figure out. It turns out that earlier in the day while Gracie was feeding the fish, she forgot to put the cap on the fish food. Don't ask how we finally figured that one out. So after half an hour of guessing, we went downstairs, put the cap on the fish food and brought it upstairs as proof. She smiled and promptly went back to sleep. It took us another hour to do the same.

The speech therapist didn't understand why I asked her to take a picture of the fish food jar with the cap off, but Elena did. We put that in the "Nighttime" section. Somehow I think we might soon have a "Wild Card" section as well.

Day 212—JUNE 28

Seven months is too short. Still, we never thought she'd make it. After being told she had 135 days to live and then later being told to expect seven months, we now have reason to celebrate. Nevertheless, seven months is too short.

I guess Elena now crosses over into undiscovered territory. As I write this, I hear of yet another child who has lost his life to this horrible disease. The cancer strikes again. And while I am happy for Elena, I am painfully aware that if she beats the average, there is another child falling victim to it. Such is the law of averages. So tonight as I hug Elena a little longer with a hint of joy in my heart, I know that the battle still awaits us, looming with uncertainty and holding no mercy.

Earlier today as Elena received her chemotherapy and I held court with the eminently qualified and compassionate team of doctors, I asked the questions I never wanted to hear myself ask. If she were to die, how would it be? Would it be peaceful? Or would it be the way I fear, the way that your mind paints a picture of it when you read other parents' accounts of their child's last moments? Of course, they never say how, but as a parent facing the same challenge, you can read between the lines. When they say, "It was a long night," you know it was more than just sleeplessness. When they say that their child had headaches, you know that it means so much more. It is a code that you never wanted to learn.

Sadly, their response was not unexpected. They said to expect breathing problems. They said it may also be nutritional or lack of fluids. They said that it may be internal bleeding. They said it may be a seizure. I didn't want the answers, but I knew I had to know. My worst fears would be much worse than reality.

Day 215—JULY 1

I'd be happy just with the porch chair swing. Brooke wants a new kitchen. Gracie wants a driveway to ride her bike on. Elena just wants it done. We all want air-conditioning. The remodeling project that started at all the wrong times drags on, partly because of my absence and always because of a lack of money. Somehow after we dug the hole and planted the foundation, cancer just wasn't in our plans. But now that it's here we're too late to stop. So we revise the project budget, do more of the projects ourselves and compromise in a battle against time.

It's not the first time we remodeled. The last time was four years ago when Elena was only two and Gracie was still curled up in Mom's arms. Back then the project was a kitchen remodel and I was just learning. To say I was unskilled labor would be a compliment. Still, it never mattered to Elena. Through it all she was right by my side offering a cookie when I was tired, a pat on the head when I hit my thumb with the hammer and praise for the finished product no matter how bad it was. The tiles were crooked, the outlets sparked and the trim was mostly caulk, but to Elena it was a work of art. Day after day, she'd sit on the bottom rung of the step stool and say, "Ohhhh, Daddy, that's pretty," as she clamped her hands together, holding them to her chest. Sometimes I'd ask her over and over again, fishing for compliments. Minutes later Brooke would walk by and laugh. "That's a bit rough," she'd say, or, "Is it supposed to leak like that?" But to Elena it was perfect.

Tonight as I build the cabinets in the new family room, I want nothing more than to hear her praise. It's not that I need it—my trim has improved, I can finally wire an outlet and I've learned to stay away from plumbing—but hearing her words would somehow mean that everything is okay. In the corner stands the step stool where she used to sit and eat cookies while I worked. After every nail I look back expecting her to be there. Meanwhile, in the next room I know she's with Brooke lying on the couch connected to an IV for fluids. It's not how I want to see my little girl and not how I ever imagined our life would turn out. I lay down the hammer. It's no longer fun without Elena.

Tomorrow I promise to build that porch chair swing. Since the very first blueprint and before we ever heard the word "cancer," I've told Elena that I would build her a porch swing so we can sit outside and talk as the sun goes down. Today that seems a distant memory as the sun sets on my daughter. The porch is nothing but framing, the concrete is hardly cured and the shingles still sit in the driveway. Still, by tomorrow night I will build that porch swing just so I can sit with her once again. Maybe we'll even have a cookie or two.

Day 216—JULY 2

Somehow I guess I never figured she would improve. After hearing from all the doctors and reading countless websites, I never once considered that she might make it. And while I occasionally posted messages of hope and positive thinking, I never really believed it would happen to us. Maybe because I was never given hope from the beginning or maybe because I was trying to protect myself from disappointment. Either way, the thought of a cure never really crossed my mind—until tonight.

I had resolved myself to soaking in the final moments. After the new chemotherapy treatment and the consequent arrival of the oxygen tanks and IV poles in the home, we figured that this was to be Elena's last treatment. But just like with everything else about this disease, it looks like we're wrong. The day started out normal, at least as normal as life gets in our home. We woke Elena by 7 A.M. and worked together to dress her and comb her hair, this time stopping four times to clean the brush of dead hair before proceeding. Then we went downstairs and attempted to feed her. But since she is only able to open her mouth less than half an inch, she is again relegated to a meal of yogurt and milk.

What was most surprising, however, is what occurred after we left for work. That's when Kelli, my cousin and a studying occupational therapist, and Grandma took over and Elena began a recovery.

The plan was to take a trip to the community all-access tree house, a tree house for children of all ages and all disabilities. We felt that this was not only an excuse to get out of the house, but also an opportunity for Elena to look at something other than the ceiling as she ate her lunch. So, packing a lunch basket, Gracie, Elena, Brooke's mother and Kelli left for the day. There I'm told that Elena ate far more than her recent staples of yogurt and milk. She ate a peanut butter cookie, some chips, a couple of blueberries and some ham and cheese. And while three months ago this would have been normal, today it was a crowning achievement. Small steps, but definitely in the right direction.

By the time I returned home from work, Elena was not only ready for dinner, but for the first time in over a month, she started to communicate through words instead of sign language. Best of all, the decision was all hers. And while the only things she said were "I want Mom to help me tomorrow morning," "I'm trying to lift my head" and "I don't want a bath," both Brooke and I knew we had made progress. She was reaching out, taking control and finally able to craft words with her previously paralyzed vocal cords. Best of all, they were sentences—not just words.

I saw Elena improve and it wasn't just because of radiation. It was because of her will and hopefully because of her treatment. And tonight, for the first time ever, I'm wondering what a cure will look like. Will she gain something every day instead of losing something? Will she get it all back or just some? How long will a recovery take? Either way, it's nice to go to bed for just one night and pray for positives rather than curse at circumstances. And while I don't want to go too far, I'll take just this moment to wonder what it can be like to have her back just like she once was.

Day 219—JULY 5

I've always felt like the kid. At least around Elena. True, I'm a lot older than she is, but for the past six years, she has been the adult, with a wisdom that transcends generations and a unique balance of emotions and common sense. Even when she was a baby, I had the sense that I was being judged by her and coached

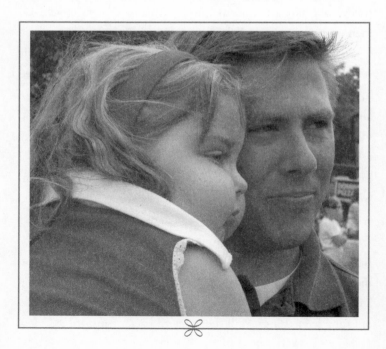

to be a better father. And let me tell you, she is an excellent coach.

From the very beginning, she taught me to say I'm sorry (mostly to Mom; sometimes I wonder if Mom had a hand in this) and to spend a little extra time with the family. Work and the chores can wait until tomorrow—family comes first. And even today, when she struggles to eat and she can't imagine walking again, she still takes a moment to improve Dad. This time she focused on my bad habit—cracking my knuckles.

This morning as I lay on the couch with her cradled in my arms, I cracked my knuckles and she moaned, looked up and placed her right hand on my finger. Shaking her head and gesturing to her own fingers, I knew what she meant. I would try, I told her. It's a nervous habit, but I will try. And I did, at least for another five minutes, as she fell asleep and I unintentionally cracked my toes within my shoes. Little did I know that I was being tested; she opened her eyes and motioned this time to my shoes. "No," she moaned, and held up her hand to signify "stop." "I understand," I told her.

Even today as Elena struggles to eat and talk, she takes the time to improve others. Ever the teacher, mom and angel, Elena is more worried about my fingers than she is about her own condition.

Day 221—JULY 7

Today I worked with Elena to get her to stand for some therapy. She responded with huffs and puffs and pouting. When I asked her if she was in pain, she said no. I asked if she was scared she would fall and she said no. I asked her why she was making such a fuss and again she shrugged. She could stand for five minutes with my help, but she just didn't want to try. For the first time, I can't connect with my daughter. I can't decipher her moods and feelings. I feel so helpless that at a time when I want to do anything and everything to make her happy, I can't find a way to do it.

Tonight Gracie found the chocolate bars my mother left behind for making s'mores. It was like gold to Elena. I haven't seen her smile that big for a long time. With each bite, she simply grinned from ear to ear. By the end of the day, we determined that we would provide chocolate therapy three times a day and research a chocolate protocol at the world-famous Hershey's Hospital. Do you think they provide it in IV formula?

Day 226—JULY 12

Therapy is a negotiation. Of course with Elena, nearly everything is. Her determination and perseverance can also translate into stubbornness when she wants them to. I guess if I went through what she has, I would be the same way. I think part of her difficulty is in having to start all over again. This is her third attempt at recovery and just as soon as she gets some of her functions back, she immediately loses them and more. She initially lost her voice and right hand. With therapy she improved, only to lose her voice, her right hand and her ability to walk. She then fought back, gaining back part of her voice and her right hand. Within months, she was able to use a walker to help her navigate the hallways of school. But now, she has lost her voice, right arm, right leg, her eyesight in her left eye and her ability to swallow and open her mouth. This time I think she's just tired of fighting.

Still, we press on and she fights us, either with a blank stare, falling to the floor or complaining of a headache.

Insert Kelli. Knowing of Elena's struggle, she bravely volunteered to help throughout the summer, giving Brooke and me a break and offering a chance to try some proven occupational techniques rather than our futile attempts at sewing cards and Play-Doh. Today, for the first time, Kelli expressed frustration with Elena's disregard for her efforts. She'd spent nights and weekends preparing creative activities and crafts, only to have Elena see through to their therapy component and refuse to participate. In a way, it is like a chess game, only Elena has you figured out before you move the first pawn.

This is the way she's always been. On trips home from school, even at four years old, she'd ask if I had any money. I would reply, "A little," and ask why. She'd ignore the question and comment on how hot it was today. "Can you wind down the window, Dad?" she'd ask. "I'm a bit hot." I'd roll down the window, immediately knowing that she had ulterior motives. Soon it would come, but only as we neared home and the local Dairy Queen. "Dad, we need to stop and get some ice cream to cool us down." There it was. Unlike any other child, who would simply ask for ice cream, Elena built her case from the time she buckled her seat belt and made sure to eliminate any excuses I might have. Did Dad have enough money? Would Dad agree it was hot? Wouldn't ice cream be the perfect solution? How could I say no? I had been outplayed.

Watching me work with Elena this afternoon, Kelli, I think,

had her doubts. Negotiating is not part of her therapy classes. I forced the issue, Elena protested with moans and screams, but in the end she did more than even Elena thought she could do: she picked up two pens and rubbed her motionless hands together. Small steps, but part of a larger path to improvement. In the end, Kelli will be better and smarter than I have been and will achieve more over the coming weeks than I have over the past months. She will harness her creativity and realize that it's okay

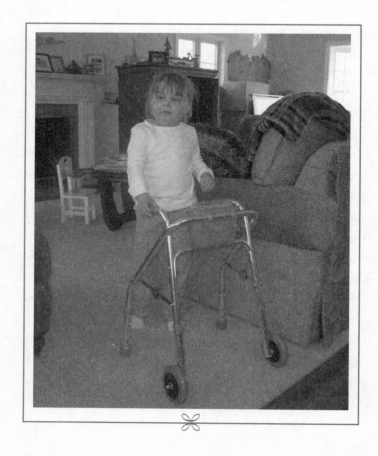

once in a while to force Elena to do more. Alternatives, rewards and creativity. All the marks of improvement. Maybe one of the rewards can be ice cream.

Day 228—JULY 14

You're not supposed to give up hope. As if the very feeling is keeping her alive. And one day you'll lose. You'll lose her.

Today hope was in short supply. I smiled when watched— the kind of smile that hides teeth tightly clenched underneath. Reality was setting in. She is not going to make it. There—I said it. But never to anyone else. Everyone tells you to keep faith and look for the cure. I can't help but be angry. And somehow I don't think I'm alone. I look in Brooke's garbage can and find just as many tissues in her can as in mine. She tries to hide them with papers, but I know the trick. I do it too.

We eat breakfast, both of us trying not to stare at her clenched hand or the teeth that barely open for even the smallest sliver of food. Still, we keep the hope. We tell her that it's much better today than yesterday. We tell her that she just needs to work her hand. We tell her that it is a matter of time. And even she knows that we're lying. She's only six years old and already too smart. Cancer ages you and after the battle she's endured Elena has the perspective of a sixty-year-old. She too has given up hope. You can tell in the million-mile stare she gives you. She's not thinking about breakfast or school. She knows too much. And somewhere I think she's trying to keep it to herself just in case we haven't figured it out yet.

Breakfasts are quiet. The day greets us coldly as we try

to find the one bright spot. But each day it gets worse. So we ignore it. We don't talk about it, we don't acknowledge it. You just don't give up hope. You just lie.

Day 229—JULY 15

I've become a daddy handkerchief and I don't mind. I have eight shirts in my drawer: five black collared ones, one blue one and two T-shirts. All of them have snot on the right shoulder. You see, now that Elena can no longer walk, we need to carry her to the kitchen table, to the bathroom and to bed. And with Brooke's bad knee, I'm the designated carrier. So picking her up from bed, I cradle her head over my right shoulder and start down the stairs. But before I can make it down the steps, Elena is blowing her nose on my shirt. What started out as a cough weeks ago has now become Elena's little joke.

Next time you see me, take a look at my right shoulder. If you're like everyone else I meet during the day, you'll comment about the white stuff on my shoulder and ask if it is paint. No. Is it drywall? No. And before you ask, all of my shirts look this way. Not only does Elena use me as a handkerchief, but now she uses my shirts as napkins too. Today my right collar has strawberry yogurt on it. No matter how many times I wash my shirt, it will always have a pink stain on the collar. I know; I've tried and will try again tonight.

In a way it's my badge; my medal of daddy service. It's also Elena's little joke. Today alone, on the way to the kitchen table, she spit out her yogurt and blew her nose twice. As I sat her down in her chair, her smile gave away her secret. This was no accident and she loved it. This was her way of getting back at Dad for all the therapy and teasing. Filling her cheeks with milk, yogurt and applesauce, she asked to use the bathroom and grinned. I knew that this was part of her plan. Looking at my shirt tonight, I was right. So the next time you see me, please excuse the shoulder. It's permanent and I can't buy enough shirts to stop it. It's Elena's little joke.

Day 230—JULY 16

Tonight my wife said the words that I didn't want to hear: "We have to at least try and make her happy while she's here." Sure, the past weeks have not been Elena's best. Her condition has taken a turn for the worse as the tumor has put its full bearing on the nerves that control her head and face. In a seemingly ironic manner, the hands that were once curled and lifeless have now regained partial function and for the first time, she possesses enough knee strength to stand with assistance while we dress her. But it is her head that we are most concerned about. Speech—even moaning—is impossible. Feeding and swallowing are tedious at best, as we struggle to nourish her with droppers and whatever amount of yogurt we can squeeze between her teeth on the tips of our fingers. The lips and tongue are motionless, left to only obstruct every chance we have at feeding her. Her eyes, which at one time served to communicate simple yeses and nos, can no longer move side to side and are fixed straight ahead, giving her permanent double vision. Worst of all, just yesterday, she lost her ability to support her own head and is now at the mercy of her unstable shoulders. Clearly this is not where we thought we'd be.

No amount of comfort can soothe Elena's sadness. No trip to Disney World or elevator ride to the top of the "Eiffel Tower" can make her happy again. She knows what we know.

Brooke's concern about Elena's happiness was normal. Her admission that Elena will not survive was not. For months, we've fought to keep hope part of our everyday lives. And although we both privately questioned her chances, we never dared discuss it between ourselves. But now, with reality casting a harsh light on our hope, it is nearly impossible to ignore. Brooke is right. And although I still plan on fighting and never once giving in, we now need to consider Elena's comfort as well as her treatment. Today we can pursue both of these goals. Someday, maybe tomorrow, we will have to choose. Sadly enough, someday may come very soon.

Day 232—JULY 18

I feel like I lived a week in only twenty-four hours. The day started with my 3:50 A.M. wake-up call as our IV fluids ran out. I wish they would give us just 100 mg more in the IV bag so I could wake at a decent hour. Unfortunately, by the time you get the first meds going and you slide back into sleep, twenty-five minutes later the alarm goes off to switch meds. An hour later, it is time to start the day. This morning was Mom's turn to stay home and the calls and visits didn't end.

That's when the phone call came in that brightened our day. We had submitted an application for a companion dog for Elena to aid her inside the house. The dog can help to alert us if Elena needs anything, as her voice has gotten too weak for us to hear if we leave the room. We didn't have much hope we would be chosen, as thousands of people need these highly trained dogs, so we figured our chances were nil. But the wonderful people recognized our urgent need, and by chance, just the right kind of dog became available as they received our application. We got the call from the organization that they could match us up and we'd be training by August 1. When I told Elena the news, I saw the first twinkle in her eyes that I had seen in a while. We made plans to shop for a toy for the dog and I explained the purpose of the dog was to help her. Elena smiled. I told her she was responsible for caring for the dog, brushing him and keeping him happy. She complained by lifting her hand, but when I assured her I would help her do this, she twinkled again.

Day 240—JULY 26

These past nine months have been a giant waiting game. We started in November when we were impatiently waiting for the bulldozers to arrive to start the home renovation. In December, we nervously waited to see results of the radiation. In January, we eagerly waited to go back to school. In February, we were endlessly waiting to go to Disney. In March, we were excitedly waiting to swim with dolphins. In May, we happily waited to see Elena's beautiful painting in the art museum. In June, we constantly waited to visit the lake in Tennessee. In July, we seem to be waiting for everything and nothing at the same time.

The girls have been waiting for their favorite friends and family to come and visit. Mom and Dad have been waiting for some peace and quiet. Elena and Gracie have been waiting for their new dog, a hope for Elena to have some control in her spinning world. Mom and Dad wait to see the smiles this new member of our family will provide. Gracie has been waiting for any free moment to go swimming. Elena has been waiting for any free moment to snuggle with Mom or Dad. We wait to see if treatments have an effect. We don't have great events or wish-granting to wait for anymore. We wait for the little things now: the smiles that a good day brings, the crazy things Gracie does to make us laugh, the small steps we take in completing our home, and the small improvements we see in Elena or the absence of decline in her condition (during progression, no decline is considered an improvement).

Life doesn't seem to just happen anymore. We don't have control of our lives; instead they are dictated by what the tumor decides to give or take away each day. I feel like I watch life coming in slow motion, while I sit and wait for it to reach me. All of a sudden I am acutely aware of every aspect of life that affects my day. It is almost like being in a hypersensitive state at all times. People talk about being pumped with adrenaline during a moment of crisis. So what happens when you are in a constant state of crisis?

Tonight, Elena called me to her bedside to tell me her left arm hurt. Most parents would give a Tylenol and send her to bed. But I can't focus my thoughts on just that arm. I think of the blood transfusions and the pages of precautions they gave us, I think of the brace and what that could do and I worry about what this problem could indicate. I finally called Keith inside, panicked by what was going on. In the end, a "medicinal" cold washcloth on the arm seemed to soothe her woes.

I wait for a time in my life when a hurt arm is just a boo-boo. When I can wake in the morning and not have to think out the entire day of medicine and feedings. Today we reversed our normal post-chemo trend of decline. Elena ate like she did the day before treatment and was awake the better part of the day begging for her cuddles. This was the day we had been waiting for. Maybe it's the waiting for the little things that keeps this uncontrollable situation slightly manageable.

Day 241—JULY 27

They were all wrong. Mom thought Elena wanted to sleep with her, not Dad. Grandma thought Elena was upset that I made her eat breakfast and lunch. Grandpa guessed that she wanted to watch TV. It was obvious that Elena was irritated and growing more frustrated by the second. Within minutes, she went from apathy to tears, and it all started when I came home from work. And knowing my reputation with Elena, everyone immediately guessed that somehow Elena did not like me. As I said, they were all wrong.

As therapy drill sergeant and mealtime dictator, Elena has never hidden her hatred for me. And ever since our final days at the hospital in early January, it was Mom who received all the love. I was good at the feedings and okay at foot massages, but Mom was the cuddler and sleeping buddy. And so, relegated to the couch, floor or Gracie's second bed, I spent the last six months waiting in the wings while Mom took center stage. Not that I minded; in my mind, anger was a form of therapy just the same. After all, if she punched me (which I encouraged her to do), she built up right-arm strength. If she was angry, at least she was active and involved. But somewhere deep inside, I missed Elena. She was always Daddy's girl for the past six years and now I had lost that as well.

When she cried this afternoon, I figured once again I was the reason. I even guessed that she wanted me to leave. But this time it was different. I asked if she wanted me to leave. Her eyes said no. I asked if she wanted me to stay. She said yes. I asked again, certain that she did not understand. And again, she said yes. I asked if she wanted me to hold her. She said yes. I asked if she was hurt and needed help. Yes again. Now we were getting somewhere. And with another five questions we had the answer. Elena wanted therapy. Elena wanted Dad. Thinking that she was mistaken, Mom asked again. Still yes. Daddy's girl was back, at least for tonight.

In the end, her back hurt and she turned to Daddy for help. And before long, with a couple of stretches, the back was feeling better and the tears had dried. I was a hero, if only for a moment. Tomorrow I think we will try a new therapy: cuddling with Dad.

Day 245—JULY 31

I've always feared that Elena would become a face of cancer, that her disease would be her identity and perhaps her legacy.

Events, tributes and memorials would soon become memories. But the longer we struggle with cancer and the more people we meet, the more we realize that we are not alone. A disease is not an identity but an obstacle. At the same time as we're fighting our own battle, we meet people who reach out to us with their battles. They have children with cerebral palsy, children who died in accidents or even their own children with cancer. And despite their pain and their struggles, they still find the time to reach out to us. This is perhaps the most telling example of all. And in a way, it is this attitude that is the true identity of the disease, the way in which you gain comfort by comforting others.

This weekend as I took Elena to the pool, I saw this first-hand. I saw her friends circle her in her wheelchair and talk to her like a friend, not like a patient. And while they asked about her new chair, her hair and why she couldn't talk, they spoke to Elena, not me. The very children who we coach on dealing with handicaps and instruct not to stare end up teaching us about caring. For to look away is to also ignore and disregard. They did neither; they asked and they cared. And Elena responded. They saw her as a friend and not as a disease.

Tonight as I look to the couch, I fear that Elena's identity is disappearing. Her left hand and foot have joined the right with partial paralysis and she now drools from the right side of her mouth. Feeding and drinking are increasingly difficult and with every passing hour, we begin to fear that these symptoms are less the result of drug side effects and more the symptoms of another progression. And so in response, we dig in with web research on our next course of action and take little comfort in the fact that there is nothing left to try. I beg for tomorrow, when she'll become her old self, and I curse myself for overreacting once again. I love those days. What do I learn from the children? Love Elena for who she is. Let the lessons and legacy come tomorrow.

Day 247—AUGUST 2

For the past nine months, she's been a pincushion. Prodded, poked and stuck. First for tests, then for treatments and now to understand her condition. And each time, she has shed a few less tears and fought back a little less. Tonight, as we relented and they inserted a feeding tube, she welcomed the change. No tears, no fight.

What started out as a quarter-inch opening between her teeth yesterday became much worse this morning when she woke up with her jaws locked closed. Two weeks ago, Mom was ready for the feeding tube; I was the holdout. I thought that the moment she had one, she'd stop fighting and give up. But tonight I realized that the battle was impossible to win and to fight it would sacrifice the very time we treasure so dearly. Still, what was most interesting was Elena's reaction. Instead of resisting, she saw the installation of a feeding tube for what it was: a way to make her life easier. Without hesitation or anticipation, she waved "yes" with her eyes and lifted her head up for the installation. And then without a tear or a flinch, she watched as they inserted the fourteen-inch tube through her nose and into her stomach.

Tonight I realize that the feeding tube will improve our days. Where we spent eight hours a day forcing food, we can now spend six hours cuddling. Still, I cannot ignore the hint of defeat in our actions and I doubt that this will improve her willingness to fight. In the end, I again find myself at the whim of consequences I cannot control but must have faith that they guide us in the right direction. For a man who believes in the power of individuals, this is not an easy realization to make. Somehow, some way, I still hope and feel that Elena will be more powerful than the cancer and smarter than the circumstances. If so, then today will be nothing more than a stop on the way to a longer and easier life.

Day 248—AUGUST 3

As I look through pictures of Elena, I'm reminded of how every trip to my mother's house involved a haircut. Sadly not one of Grandma's haircuts ever looked good. Crooked bangs, uneven sides; sometimes I wondered what my mother was thinking. Each trip her hair would get shorter and shorter until her bangs would disappear, leaving only a few crooked hairs remaining.

It never really mattered to Elena.

Seven months later she now begins her decline and has lost even the pink highlights as a result of the chemotherapy. And for a girl who loved her hair, this was not easy. Her hair makes her feel pretty and healthy. Even after Grandma's haircuts, it would grow back again ready for the next day they would spend together. Brooke and I would cringe; Grandma and Elena would laugh. A day at the salon—Grandma's way.

Day 249—AUGUST 4

Walk slowly. Throw petals. Don't step on your dress. Don't move, and be quiet. All the essentials of flower girl etiquette and Gracie knew them well. "I know, I know. Walk slow. Throw petals. Don't step on my dress. Don't move, and be quiet," she'd

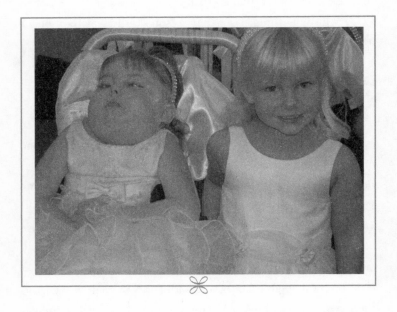

say on the way to the wedding, on the walk to the church and while she stood in line ready to enter the sanctuary. Who told her these things we have no idea, but apparently our advice wasn't necessary; someone had gotten to her before we had.

Today was Kelli and John's wedding. (Okay, it's always the bride's wedding. The groom is just along for the ride.) Kelli was Elena's caregiver this summer, and her wedding was something

Elena had looked forward to for the past three months. Personally I think Elena was a shoe-in for the flower girl position all
along. Gracie, thankfully, was also included to make our lives
easier. But that didn't keep Gracie from stealing the show.

This was Elena and Gracie's first opportunity at flower girl
status. And somewhere in the spectrum of little-girl honors, this
falls no more than two steps below princess. Needless to say, the
dress was picked out early, even before Kelli's announcement, in
preparation for yet another wedding (her aunt's wedding, which
is in less than a month). And in the mass hysteria of wedding-
palooza that will rock our family this year, it was decided that
the girls would wear the dresses of their choice, as long as they
wore white. That way, they could go with any color in the wedding party. So in accordance with bridal protocol, Gracie picked
out a white dress with pink flowers, and Elena chose a completely
pink dress with ruffles. So much for wedding protocol. But who
was going to tell Elena no? What Elena wants, Elena gets. Kelli
chose green for her bridesmaids' gowns. Her flowers were red
and white. Even the men wore green cummerbunds. Still, Elena
wore pink.

In the days before the wedding, the air was thick with anticipation. Plans were made and rehearsed. Dresses were inspected
daily. Every little detail was obsessed over. For Elena, the night
before was a sleepless one. Somehow, I think Kelli slept better.
Elena is a girl who stacks her books according to size and color
on her bookshelf, and we once again saw the obsessive habits rise
to the surface. I never thought I would be as pleased as I was to
see them again. Finally she cared about something other than
sleeping with Mom that night.

From my mother to Aunt Jenny and Aunt Jackie, everyone seemed eager for Elena's big premiere. And while we worried that Kelli's wedding would soon become Elena's flower girl presentation, it was Kelli who also went out of her way to encourage Elena's participation. I don't know if this was intended as a distraction for Elena or just an excuse for ceremony, but for this we are eternally grateful. It's not too often that you get to see your daughters walking down the aisle. Even once is enough for any father.

By evening's end, the wedding had gone off without a hitch. Elena was attentive and excited. Even with her paralysis, we could tell through her eyes with every "yes" and "no" nod. For her part, Gracie walked slowly, stayed off her dress and threw petals. So many, as a matter of fact, that by the time she reached the seventh pew, she had dispensed the majority of petals and the rear of the sanctuary resembled a rose slaughter. This did not prevent her from throwing imaginary petals in their place. As I said before, she stole the show once again.

Today was a welcome relief from the events of the past week. At every step, we've tried to encourage Elena and coax even a hint of her personality from her lips or eyes. But with paralysis now affecting everything other than her eyes, we have received no such sign. And so begin the inevitable thoughts as you see her close herself off from the rest of the world, as she no longer reacts to even the most loving touch or your good-night kiss. It's then as a father that you begin to wonder if she's really there. Does she know what you whisper in her ear, does she know that you're holding her hand? Or are you inserting this feeding tube and continuing these IVs for your benefit and not hers? And what about quality of life? Or is that just a fancy way of giving up the fight while rationalizing your true intentions away? And if you do give up, will you say one day it was for the best, while wondering secretly what would have happened if you were stronger and had kept up the fight? I do not profess to know these answers, nor do I think I want to hear them from someone else. Still, after a week of seeing no response, I wonder if this is what makes it easier to stop the fight. Had I already lost my Elena when she stopped responding a week ago? And while I know that thinking, feeling girl still resides under that lifeless face, what is life without communication? Oh, how I needed a sign from her tonight.

Tonight I would learn how little I knew. Through the wedding, she finally responded with excitement and passion. In her eyes, Brooke and I saw her watch, wonder and dream of a wedding of her own. Complete with flower girls and her own white flowing dress (or possibly pink). Still, it was at the reception that we finally communicated, this time as a daughter and her dad.

As we sat watching the girls twirl with abandonment on the empty dance floor, spinning themselves endlessly and then falling to the floor, Elena motioned to me with her eyes. Did she need to use the bathroom? No. Did she want a pretzel? No. Was she uncomfortable? No. Was she cold? No. I was out of questions. So we sat, quietly watching Gracie twirl and fall once more, this time laughing all the way down. Did she want to dance? I asked. "Yes," she nodded. Did she want to twirl? No. Did she want to dance with Mom? No. I paused. She never before wanted to cuddle with Dad. She never wanted Dad's comfort at the doctor's office. She never even wanted Dad to tickle her before bed. Still,

I asked, "Do you want to dance with Dad?" "Yes," she nodded enthusiastically. I asked again. Obviously she must have misunderstood, but the answer was still the same.

One song. Two songs. A third song and finally a fourth. Through it all, she kept nodding yes and asking for more. This was Dad's dance and no one was about to take it away from me. It was the dance I had always wanted, just not at the wedding I expected. So there on an empty dance floor to Lionel Ritchie songs that I was sure the DJ must have gotten for free at some garage sale, we danced with Gracie, Allyson and Michelle, twirl-

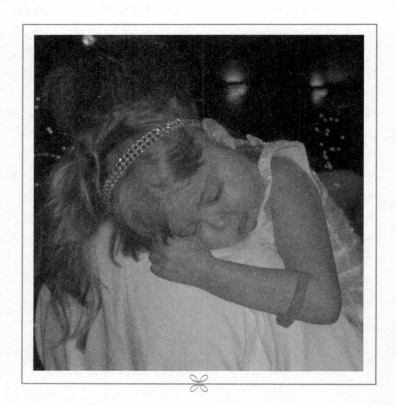

ing until dizzy. My dancing was shoddy, the atmosphere was less than perfect, but it was a night I will never forget. And by the third song, I slowly felt her hand open from its paralytic clenched fist and move to pat my neck. Communication. Not by words and not by eyes, but by love. I pray one day to get that dance again, this time at her very own wedding.

Day 250—AUGUST 5

Wake up early. Eat two bowls of breakfast. Play fetch with the dog. Go for a walk with the family. Visit more family. Read five books. Go to bed. For any normal child, this would be a full day. For Elena, it was nothing short of miraculous.

After spending the past three weeks unable to open her mouth even enough to sip milk, Elena began the day without restrictions. Hinting that she was hungry the moment she woke up, we jumped at the opportunity to try to feed her without the help of the feeding tube still hanging from her nostril. Never mind that she had already eaten the equivalent of a day's worth of calories through the tube since the moment she went to sleep last night; she was still hungry. And when we found out that her teeth had finally relinquished their viselike grip, we knew we were in for a day of surprises. Quickly, we pushed everything we could find in the freezer into her awaiting mouth before it could close and disappear forever. Thankfully her mouth cooperated as she not only inhaled a cup of yogurt, but also a few pretzels, some strawberries, some cereal and two glasses of milk over the course of the day.

From there, it was nothing but pure excitement as we

watched our daughter blossom once again, complete with her obsessive intentions and her drive to be normal. Her paralysis started to fade with an occasional lift of her head and a motion with her left hand. Surely even she could be satisfied with her progress over one day. So when we found her crying at the dinner table at her grandpa-grandpa's house, we were puzzled. It turned out that to her, part of being normal was also playing in the backyard with Gracie and the other kids. And so, lifting the wheelchair in our arms, we carried her on her throne down the deck stairs to the waiting game in the yard below. And although no one kept score, we all knew who had won that day.

Tonight as we put the girls to bed, we recapped today's successes while reading our favorite collection of knock-knock joke books. The punch lines weren't new and the jokes were clean, but to Elena and Gracie, it was a wonderful way to end the day. Gracie would begin with the "Knock-knock," to which Elena would respond with eye blinks to spell out each syllable of "Who's there?" and "Archie who?" Even Pueblo, our new resident canine sibling, joined in with the occasional bark to prod Elena along when she fell off to sleep. And by the time Gracie delivered the punch line, funny or not, we all laughed, including Elena.

"Knock-knock."
"Who's there?"
"Sue."
"Sue who?"
"SURPRISE!!!"

Yes, definitely a surprise and a very special one. Let's do it again tomorrow.

Day 254—AUGUST 9

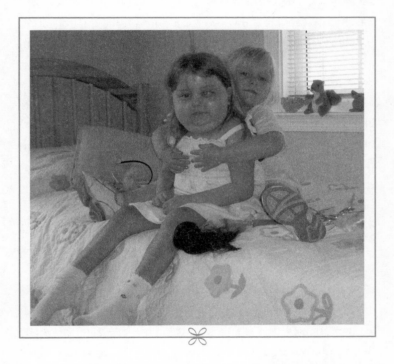

I fear that Elena knows more than we do. Over the past three days, she has asked to dance with Dad, play in the backyard, eat a Happy Meal and chocolate ice cream, go swimming, take a bath and play a card game. But what's more interesting than her sudden burst of energy has been the fact that for the past several months, she's shunned each and every one of these activities. She chose Dad over Grandma and Mom as her dance partner, the same man she spurned when it came time to cuddle, eat or sleep. She wanted to play a game she never played before, a game in which her paralyzed arms would prove useless. She wanted a Happy Meal, despite knowing that she could never even eat the smallest fry. For her, just the sight of it was enough. She asked for chocolate ice cream, which for a pure vanilla girl was nothing short of astonishing. She actually asked to go swimming, an activity that she came to fear as she began to lose the use of her arms in early January. She wanted to take a bath, despite her recent fear of any activity that might result in the loss of more hair. And finally, yesterday, she wanted to play a card game. She never really enjoyed a game of cards. To tell you the truth, neither did I, but it was something to distract us as we passed the day from waiting room to waiting room. To both of us, it came to represent everything we hated about hospital life.

Together these activities symbolize everything that Elena either feared or never did. And for three days, she was well enough to experience it all. She could finally open her mouth, move her left hand and communicate with us through blinks of her eyes. But this morning, all of that stopped. The hand is again motionless, the mouth is limp and her left eye is completely blind and paralyzed. She feeds from her feeding tube and drinks from her IV. And now our vital link of communication with our daughter has been severed. What was once three days of celebration now has the potential to be our best and final memories.

Today we made another trip to the emergency room. Brooke and I hold Elena's hands as we watch her chest rise and fall with every breath. We've been here before and pray for the opportunity to do it over again. But as I hear her breathe from across the room with a whine and hesitation, I realize that somehow, this time, it is different. My little girl, who has surprised so many and stolen life from this tumor four times before at the last moment, no longer has protocols, treatments or antibiotics to help her. It is up to her and we can only stand by and watch. Tonight will be a long night. I now know that she knows more than we do; I just pray that she also has the courage and will to match.

Day 255—AUGUST 10

There's something about the inevitable. Tonight the inevitable is all we have. No longer do we have the medicines, the chemotherapy or control over our own lives—we are powerless. Powerless as we grapple with Elena's sickness. Powerless as we sit by her side holding her hand. Powerless as we watch her struggle to breathe.

Tonight Elena began the inevitable. After an hour of opening her eyes this morning, she slowly succumbed and fell into a coma. And for what seemed like a lifetime, we watched each individual breath as she hesitated and coughed. And for the first time, both Brooke and I realize the struggle has been lost. I guess that happens during a coma. When the last thread of communication is lost and the distance begins. The distance between Gracie and Elena. The distance between Elena and us. The distance between her and a cure. The memories start to fade as our hopes turn toward a painless end for our brave little girl.

For the past seven months we've watched and waited for our turn. Watching as child after child became a statistic. Knowing the end and how it would come. Now we wonder.

Day 256—AUGUST 11

Today we know what it's like. The empty feeling, the one that cannot be pacified and aches to be filled. Last night as Elena fell into a coma and her breathing became short, we decided to finally tell Gracie about what lay ahead. So there, in the backyard on the steps of Elena's playhouse that I built for the girls, we told Gracie that her sister was going to die. We explained that Elena was going to be an angel in heaven. And tonight she would have to say good-bye. Gracie, in her own fashion, asked if Elena would get wings and then suggested that we bring Elena out so she could show her her rock collection.

The rest of the evening was spent by the playhouse with Elena struggling to breathe and our entire family around to comfort her. And with Brooke to her right and me on her left, we held her hands under the tree she helped us plant when we first moved to our new house. It was her tree, her choice: a brilliant scarlet maple.

Throughout the night she was at peace. At times, she strained to breathe under the pressure of the tumor, but through it all she continued to sleep. Brooke and I lay by her side in bed until early this morning, when she finally relented and left us.

Today Gracie has remaining questions and so do we. I'm sure all will be answered in time, but not by any person and not today. All that remains is our love for our daughters and our desire to remember Elena free of cancer. The house is now quiet and so are our hearts.

This morning I carried Elena in my arms to the waiting ambulance. She is still my daughter and I know she would appreciate being carried in my arms rather than being placed on a stretcher. She will continue to be our daughter and a part of our family forever. And although all traces of medical supplies and equipment were set outside our door within hours, her pictures will always grace our walls as a reminder of the inspiration she was to all of us.

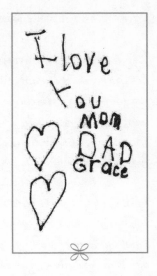

In the end, we decided on an autopsy to garner any information about this tumor in the hopes of helping other children afflicted with this hopeless disease. We pray and will work to continue Elena's fight in pursuit of a cure and make sure that her life continues to inspire long beyond today. The service and tributes will come later.

For today, the memories and tears continue. We now sit at a table for three, and in the backseat of a car as a family. The bed isn't as small as it once was and our house is too large. And in our hearts we are reminded by notes hidden throughout the house over the past nine months by Elena: "I love you Mom, Dad and Grace." We love you too, Elena. More than you can possibly imagine.

After Elena, Day 1—AUGUST 12

Today we ache. Elena's favorite stuffed animals, her dresses and her sparkly shoes remain in her closet untouched. We can't make it through even a sentence without pausing to reflect. Where we once said "Come on, girls," we now have to stop and say "Gracie." It's amazing how even the smallest pronouns make you stop and wonder what could have been.

I mourn now. I guess I was so busy putting on a strong image to Elena that I never bothered to consider death as a reality. Sure, I questioned why and wondered about the extent of her will to fight, but deep down I ignored every urge to confront it. Now I can barely make it through an hour without holding a picture tight or making a trip to her room to remember. I guess I just don't want to forget. The sight of her beautiful eyes, her long eyelashes, the sound of her sweet voice and the smell of her hair.

Last night as the sun faded from view and the last visitor left our driveway, we sat as a family of three on the front step and looked to the horizon. In the parting moments of the sunset, pink clouds covered the sky. Gracie was the first to make the connection. "Look, Mom, Elena's clouds," she said. She was right. And so for the final minutes of daylight, we were a family of four once again. Pink was always her favorite color. Thanks for the show, Elena.

After Elena, Day 3—AUGUST 14

At night they looked like angels. Lost in a dream, quiet and peaceful. And I wanted nothing more than one last look at the two girls that meant so much to me. So tiptoeing into their room

I would turn off the night-light, cover them with the quilt that had been tossed aside moments before and kiss them good night. But before leaving, I would always lean over and whisper into their ears, "You are my princess. You are smart, you are pretty and you will do amazing things." I would softly stroked their hair before retiring to our room at the end of the hall.

With me, there was never any doubt. Elena and Gracie may have needed the reminder, but I knew that my daughters would always achieve where I had failed. They would stand on the shoulders of my family before them and accomplish the impossible. And Brooke and I would stand on the sidelines and be their biggest fans.

The day Elena died, our world was shattered. She and her sister would always be my princesses. They would be smart and they were certainly pretty. But Elena had only six short years, certainly not enough to do amazing things. Tonight I know I am wrong. In six years she accomplished the impossible and she succeeded where I had failed. Only this time, her role was to inspire, and the journey was to be made by others. I see this not only in the efforts of people everywhere coming together to cure cancer, but more directly in the letters that we still receive that start with "You don't know me but . . . ," and then continue on to tell me how their lives were changed by her struggle to simply live.

Elena's lesson is not one of death and cancer; instead it is one of hope and life. She taught me how to live, how to love and how to laugh. I will never forget that lesson.

Tonight I continue to stroke Gracie's hair and whisper into her ear, "You are my princess. You are smart, you are pretty and you will do amazing things." I know she will. But before I leave her room, I touch the picture of Elena that hangs above the light switch and whisper, "I love you, Elena. You will accomplish amazing things."

After Elena, Day 4—AUGUST 15

Yesterday morning I received a call from the chaplain of the hospital. Elena's remains had been cremated and she wanted to personally deliver them. It's funny. Throughout the entire process, I always thought this would be the moment I would dread the most. I had envisioned that when I held her ashes, I would come to the realization that she was really gone—forever. Instead, I was relieved to have her home once again. It's not that her body holds any true significance; her soul is always with us. Still, her body was a tangible symbol of what was left of my daughter and I wanted to have her back home. Carrying her to the ambulance after her death was the hardest. For the first time in her short life, she was in someone else's hands. Minute after minute, I'd wonder where she was. It permeated my thoughts and invaded my nights as I worried about her body, all the while wishing that somehow she would come home soon. Finally, she did.

Then I was left with a pewter canister containing her ashes. Small, cold and simple. Nothing like my daughter, but I still couldn't make myself let go. I sat on the couch and held it in my arms for what seemed like hours. Somehow you never think this will happen to your daughter. I envisioned holding her in the palms of my hands as an infant, cradling her as a toddler, consoling her as a child, hugging her as a teenager and walking her down the aisle as a young woman. But never did I think I would hold her in this manner.

Brooke and I decided long ago to spread Elena's ashes; no urn and no burial. In our minds, this was the only way to continue. Simple ceremony; Mom, Dad and Gracie. Elena, in all of her humility, would have preferred her ashes to be placed close to home. So looking to the backyard, we found our answer.

Three years ago, Elena was barely three years old. Gracie was still on Mom's hip. We had just moved into the house and knew that a remodeling project was imminent. But with no money, all we could do was plant trees. Besides that, if we planted trees now, by the time we were ready to remodel they would be mature and help shade the yard. We picked an ash, a willow, an oak, a sugar maple and a magnolia. Partly a product of budget and partly because we figured that with more diversity, we were guaranteed that something would grow, we planted trees that didn't necessarily match. When Elena suggested that we also buy a pink dogwood, we figured that we'd better stop while we were ahead. "No," we told her. It would never survive the deer that raid our backyard every night. Still, Elena pressed. "How about a red one?" she asked. Okay, she wanted a tree, so be it. So slogging back through the mud at the nursery we picked a scarlet maple. At least two of the trees would match and this way it would at least be green most of the year. The tree was scrawny, but it was also cheap. So we bought it, never expecting it to survive or flourish. Three years later, it's the strongest tree in the yard and also the prettiest. Still, fall after fall, it never turns red. Instead, it turns burnt orange two days before dropping its leaves.

Tomorrow, Elena's tree will also become her final resting place. In preparation, we built a stone fence around the bed and planted pink mums in her honor. I only pray that I am strong enough to let her go when we release her ashes there tomorrow. And maybe this fall, the tree will finally turn scarlet red, but knowing Elena, I wouldn't be surprised if it is pink.

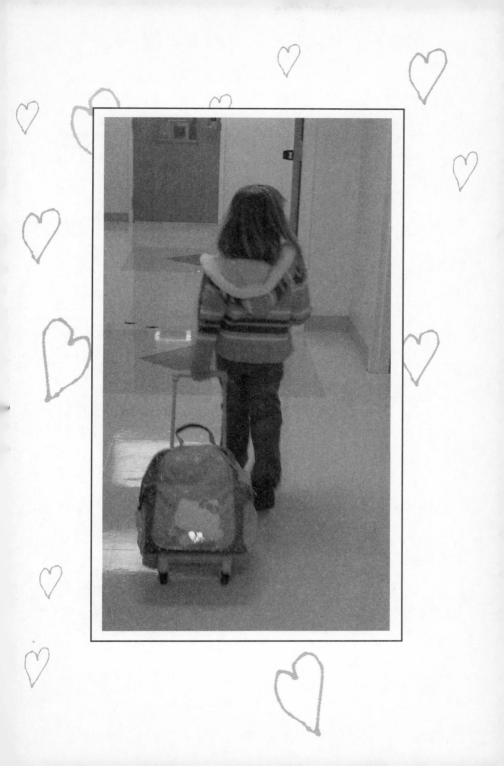

afterword

ALTHOUGH I CAN'T remember every moment of her life, I can remember the nights. Nights started with a bath and a book. She'd always choose the biggest book and we'd always beg for the simple one. Somehow we'd always settle on *A Light in the Attic* or *One Fish, Two Fish, Red Fish, Blue Fish.* We'd read and she would listen, but as the book dragged on and we would skip a page, she would catch us and turn the page back. What I wouldn't give to have those pages back. Then we'd end the night with a kiss, a tickle and a comment of how proud we were. Those are the nights I'd love to relive.

They say that it gets easier over time. That one day you begin to accept her death. In truth I don't think I ever will. Instead, you come to treasure the simpler moments of life and in doing so you find peace. In Elena's case, she was the teacher and lessons she left behind are wrapped in pink heart-shaped notes hidden throughout the house. She alone taught us to be better people and a stronger family than we could ever imagine.

Since her death, the lessons remain strong, but so do the emotions. Every moment and every action is a reminder of her legacy. Still, each and every day, Elena remains part of our family. Her pictures still grace our walls and her inspiration lives on today in the actions of her charity. And with this, we will never forget.

Today Gracie has a wisdom that I wish she never had. Brooke and I have perspective. What was once critical is now trivial and what once was a priority is a distraction. We are fearless. Death is merely part of life rather than an ending, and what it brings is value and focus to what we see as important. Every day, we see life as a gift and every moment as an opportunity. And we do so because Elena has taught us the most valuable lesson of all.

One day we'll pass this lesson on to Gracie through the pages of this journal. Most of it she'll already know. But perhaps it might teach her to love her own children, tickle them as they run off to bed and never skip a page. I hope so. It's Elena's lesson and one I'll never forget.

the cure starts now

ELENA IS NOT ALONE. Every day thousands are faced with cancer. Many will survive. Too many will die. In many ways this book is a message to us all, written with the intention of preserving the memories of one six-year-old girl for her sister, who is too young to remember. Still, if it has any effect, perhaps it will teach us all how to treasure those moments with our loved ones and learn the true value of life.

This book also has another message. In writing to Gracie on March 3 we ended the journal with one simple message: the cure starts now. To us it was a pledge—a decision to not accept cancer and never succumb. Death and suffering at the hands of this disease is not inevitable and not "God's will." We, as parents, could do more. In time it was adopted as a motto by family and friends. Today it is a cause that offers new hope and direction in the form of a nonprofit organization. Now it is a calling that we, as a society, can do more.

In fighting cancer we have two strategies. Currently we only fight with one. Most often we fight cancer by the numbers. We run survey after survey predicting fatality rates and then prioritize funding research according to how many people die. It is a strictly political strategy for a worldwide disease that knows no political boundaries. It is a comfortable strategy—even reasonable to some—but still, it should never be our only one. Year after year, more people die and the organizations leading the fight celebrate anniversaries in excess of seventy years or more. Let us as a society find it unacceptable that the fight cannot be won and that it should take decades to cure what we should have cured decades ago.

There is a second strategy. It is neither politically friendly nor easy. It is about targeting those cancers that offer us the most to learn. Some of these cancers affect thousands of people, others affect few, but regardless of their magnitude, the lessons we may learn may cure us all. Pediatric brain cancer is a cancer that we can all learn from. It may also give us a "home run" cure for cancer if we can apply its lessons universally to all cancers. So in curing cancer, starting with our children may be the smartest strategy of all. And in doing so we may be ensuring that twenty years from now the fight is over for good.

This "home run" strategy for cancer is not without its difficulties. It is not an alternative to the strategy of curing cancer by the numbers, but it is worthy of our attention and our funding. But unlike other cancer strategies, our support may never come from a governmental budget or policy. Instead it will come from you.

In the end, it will start with children like my daughter Elena. Soon it will become a movement. One day it might become a cure for us all. Our children deserve better. The Cure Starts Now.

To learn more about The Cure Starts Now,
the children we celebrate and the organization Elena inspired,
visit www.thecurestartsnow.org.

acknowledgments

WE STARTED THIS journey alone as a family of four, only to be joined along the way by family, friends and strangers who shared the inspiration left by Elena and made it their own. Without their love and support we would have been lost. We are forever grateful.

Thank you also to our family and friends for their support and influence in the publishing of this book. In addition, we are grateful for the devotion of our agent, Sharlene Martin; the guidance of our publicist, Justin Loeber; and the dedication of Lisa Sharkey, Amy Kaplan and the entire HarperCollins team. Their patience, integrity and dedication to Elena's legacy comforted us in ways we never thought possible and helped us overcome our fears of publishing this journal. We would also like to offer a special thank-you to Martha Montgomery, Patricia Harman, Judy Morgan and Margaret Theile for their efforts in clarifying Elena's message from online journal to paper. And always, to Tiffany Kinzer, who insisted that this book be more than just for Gracie.